Arms Wide Open

Arms Wide Open

A Midwife's Journey

Patricia Harman

BEACON PRESS, BOSTON

Beacon Press
25 Beacon Street
Boston, Massachusetts 02108-2892
www.beacon.org

Beacon Press books
are published under the auspices of
the Unitarian Universalist Association of Congregations.

14 13 12 11   8 7 6 5 4 3 2 1

This book is printed on acid-free paper that meets the uncoated paper ANSI/
NISO specifications for permanence as revised in 1992.

Text design by Wilsted & Taylor Publishing Services

Library of Congress Cataloging-in-Publication Data
Harman, Patricia.
Arms wide open : a midwife's journey / Patricia Harman.
p. ; cm.
ISBN 978-0-8070-0138-7 (hardcover : alk. paper)
1. Harman, Patricia, 1943– 2. Midwives—United States—Biography. I. Title.
[DNLM: 1. Harman, Patricia, 1943– 2. Nurse Midwives—Personal Narratives.
3. Midwifery—Personal Narratives. WZ 100]
RG950.H357 2008
618.20092—dc22
[B]
2010034526

To my best friend, Tom,
and to all those idealists
who believe there is a better way

Midwife—to be with women at childbirth and throughout life

AUTHOR'S NOTE

Arms Wide Open: A Midwife's Journey is based on journals I kept for many years. The events were recorded in detail, but there are gaps, and I painted in those gaps to the best of my recollection. All the characters, except my husband, Tom Harman, have been disguised, to protect their privacy. The patients described are composites, based on real people.

Arms Wide Open is not just for those interested in midwifery or feminism. It's for anyone, of any gender, young or old, who cares about the earth and social justice. We each have our own song. This is mine and I sing it for you.

All the way down Route 119, past Gandeeville, Snake Hollow, and Wolf Run, I'm thinking about the baby that died.

I wasn't there, didn't even know the family. It happened a few days ago, with another midwife, at a homebirth in Hardy County, on summer solstice, the longest day of the year.

Word on the informal West Virginia midwives' hotline is that the baby's shoulders got stuck, a grave emergency. The midwife, Jade, tried everything, all the maneuvers she'd studied in textbooks and the special tricks she'd learned from other practitioners, but nothing worked. They rushed, by ambulance, to the nearest hospital thirty miles away, with the baby's blue head sticking out of the mother, but it was too late. Of course it was too late.

Homebirth midwives in West Virginia are legal, but just barely, and there's no doubt the state coroner's office will investigate. Jade is afraid. We are all afraid.

We whip around another corner and I lose my supper out the side window. *Who do I think I am taking on this kind of responsibility? Why am I risking my life to get to a homebirth of people I hardly know? What am I doing in this Ford station wagon being whipped back and forth as we careen through the night?*

༝

I awake sick with grief, my heart pounding. I'm lying on a pillow-pad-ded king-size bed with floral sheets. A man I hardly recognize sleeps next to me. This is Tom, I remind myself: my husband of thirty-three years, a person whose body and mind are as familiar to me as my own. I prop myself up on an elbow, inspecting his broad shoulders, smooth face, straight nose and full lips, his short silver hair, in the silver moon-light. One hairy leg sticks out of the covers. One arm, with the wide hand and sensitive surgeon's fingers, circles his pillow. It's 3:45, summer solstice morning.

When I rise and pull on my long white terry robe, I stand for a moment, getting my bearings, then open the bedroom door that squeaks and pad across the carpeted living room. Outside the tall corner windows, the trees dance in the dark. Once I called myself Trillium Stone. That was my pen name when I lived in rural communes, wrote for our political rag, *The Wild Currents*, taught the first natural-childbirth classes, and started doing homebirths.

Now I'm a nurse-midwife with short graying hair, who no longer delivers babies, living with an ob-gyn in this lakefront home, so far from where I ever thought I would live, so far from where I ever *wanted* to live. I search the photographs on the piano of my three handsome sons, now men. Do I wake? Do I sleep?

OK, my life has been a wild ride, I'll admit it, but the image of this hippie chick lurching through the night, on her way to a homebirth, with only a thick copy of *Varney's Midwifery* as a guide, disturbs me. What did she think she was doing? Where did she get the balls?

🜨

On the highest shelf in the back of our clothes closet, a stack of journals gathers dust. For seventeen years I carried them in a backpack from commune to commune. They've moved with me across the country three times, through midwifery school, Tom's medical school and his ob-gyn residency. I can't get the diaries out of my mind, a mute witness to my life . . .

I slip back through the bedroom. Tom snores on. By the dim closet light, I find a stepladder and struggle to bring down the shabby container. The journals have been closed for twenty-five years; pages stick together and smell faintly of mold.

I'm on a mission now, trying to understand, but I'm surprised to find that I started each entry with only the day and the month, no year. This is going to take a while. It seems I never expected anyone would want to reconstruct my life, not even me. I'm an archaeologist digging through my own past.

With narrowed eyes, I flip through notebook after notebook, daring that flower child to show her face. When the alarm goes off, Tom, dressed in blue scrubs for the OR, finds me asleep in the white canvas chair, with a red journal open, over my heart.

FROM THE RED JOURNAL

❧

Little Cabin in the North Woods

1971–1972

❧

Fall

CHAPTER I

Home

"Keep up," Stacy yells into a bitter wind, turning to wait for me. "This kid is getting heavy." In the dim light, I can just see his face, his narrow nose, his long eyelashes, his brown beard and brown hair, a dark Scot with a square jaw and the back of an ox. He has the baby carrier on his back and a heavy canvas backpack loaded with supplies on his front. I try to pick up my pace, but I, too, am carrying a large knapsack of provisions, and though I'm sturdy and big boned, I'm not as strong as my lover.

The swamp is damp with second-growth cedars that lean close like old women. We squish along the narrow path until we come to the creek and find it flooded. To get home, we must cross on unstable logs. Stacy goes first with one-year-old Mica. I trudge behind, after finding a long stick to balance myself. One wrong move and I'll tumble into the water.

The trip to Duluth was a disappointment. We'd hiked out of the homestead and then hitched into town, but three out of four friends we went to see were in Minneapolis at a war resisters' meeting. I sigh into the dark.

Sometimes I'm tired of this difficult life, living without electricity, running water, indoor plumbing, or a vehicle, but it's my choice. No one is forcing me to live in a two-room log cabin, on a remote farm, a mile from the nearest dirt road, ten miles from the closest store.

We traverse the big meadow where we have our garden and wind through the balsam grove, along the path to the smaller clearing. In the fading light, our two-story log house, taller than it is wide, looms over us. As always when we come up to it through the trees, its solid bulk surprises me. We built this cabin, overlooking the Lester River, with our own hands. It is ours and we are home.

Repentance

Rain, rain, a snare drum on the roof. All morning it rains and we work inside, chinking. Once, this hundred-year-old Finnish log house sat rotting on our friend Jason's Christmas tree farm. Last summer we deconstructed it, hauled it ten miles over dirt roads on a borrowed logging truck, planed the old surface down to new wood, built a foundation, and reassembled the timbers like Lincoln Logs. It was grueling, hot work, with mosquitoes buzzing over our heads, but I loved it . . .

Mica crawls on the floor in his corduroy coveralls, plays in the wood chips. When he starts to fuss, I stop chinking and nurse him. Stacy has gone upstairs to take a nap. That's one thing I appreciate about living here. You can sleep when you want to, work when you want to, make love when you want to. No time clocks. No boss constantly watching over you.

From my perch on the window seat, I gaze out the window. The Lester River, sixty feet down the grassy slope, is up to its banks. White foam floats on the water. Wildflowers encircle us, goldenrod and deep purple aster. A flock of yellow finch swoops down on the blossoms, looking for seeds. Except for this clearing and the five-acre meadow where we garden, uninhabited forest surrounds us for miles.

One year old, Mica pulls my long braids while he nurses. I caress his fine white cobweb hair. This is the first time Stacy and I have lived alone as a couple, and it isn't something we aspired to. When we bought this land two summers ago and still lived at Chester Creek House, an urban commune, our friends seemed interested in establishing a rural outpost. So far it's just us. I'm not sure I mind; I feel safer out in the woods. There's less risk I'll run into Johan, less chance I'll shatter the delicate balance of my nuclear family, crack it open like a blue robin's egg.

It wasn't supposed to happen. I never meant it to happen. The whole beautiful, sordid business is a paragraph in someone else's life.

We were living at the Draft Counseling Center in Duluth, on Third Street, helping conscientious objectors and hiding the occasional draft evader on his way to Canada. This was after we left Freefolk, a small commune near Bemidji, Minnesota. Stacy was taking welding classes at the vocational school and I was four months pregnant, on purpose, with our baby.

While Stacy was at class during the day, Johan Sorensen and I talked about peace and the revolution. He gave me shoulder rubs and then back rubs. Then my neck . . . I never hid that we were sexually involved. I was single, though the seed of new life grew inside me.

Stacy and I didn't believe in marriage . . . Still, my unfaithfulness wounded him, cut him deep. I try not to think about it. It's better with just the three of us here.

When Mica was born, everything changed. My sacrifice on the altar of birth burned some of the selfishness out of me. I was a mother now and even I couldn't handle three males in my life.

❦

I gently lay my sleeping baby down on the window seat, touch the little brown birthmark near his ear, tuck a blanket around him, and study the yellow-poplar log walls. The Finnish pioneer who originally built this dwelling fit the timbers so tight you can't see daylight, but still wind whistles through. If we don't finish chinking by snowfall, we'll have to move back to town. I stand and maneuver another piece of firewood into the cookstove.

❦

The rain stops and as the low sun slants golden under the clouds, Stacy clomps down the stairs. I see first, in the shaft of light that comes in from the window, his narrow bare feet and then his jeans and finally his whole, powerful, shirtless body.

Here is a man who loves work and music and movement and sex. Here is a man who would walk through fire to halt injustice or save a child. He leans forward and peers out the window, where each drop of water at the end of each balsam needle reflects the fading day. "Want to go out for a walk?" he asks.

The fire crackles in the woodstove. How could I want anything more?

Alone

Three days of intermittent cold rain and then the low, flat gray clouds move on. The sky is clear, but by afternoon the light fades. Already we've had a hard frost. Stacy sits on the stairs, tying his boots. He's on his way out to our mailbox at the end of Dahl Road.

"Wait just a second; I want you to take my letter for Colin." As I rummage around in the tin box where we keep the stamps, I glance at our money jar on the same shelf. Almost empty.

"Do you really want to walk all that way? It'll be night soon. You could wait until morning."

"No, I'm up for a hike. I need the exercise." Stacy shuts the heavy oak door behind him and I can hear the Big Ben alarm clock ticking upstairs.

All day we've been chinking, slow and tedious work. Outside there's more chinking to do and more tasks. The window over the kitchen table is still covered with plastic. We need to dig a pit for the root crops and get in more firewood before snow. Winter comes early in the North Woods.

I stare out the corner window at the darkening day. Weathermen bombings, the Manson murders, and Ronald Reagan's announcement, as the governor of California, "If it takes a bloodbath, let's get it over with," have eroded hippie popularity.

Everywhere there is craziness with drugs and cops and demonstrations gone bad. In the Victorian house on Haight Street in San Francisco, where I lived after I dropped out of Lewis & Clark College, there was a jar of peyote buttons on the mantel and strangers shooting up in the kitchen. We could see that our utopian dream was turning into a nightmare and left early to build the new world elsewhere.

A few years ago, people waved at us when we strolled down the street; found us interesting, exotic birds blown in from some other continent. Long-haired hippie women with flowers behind their ears smiled on the cover of *Time*.

The last time Stacy and I hitched to town, car after car passed us by, the drivers averting their eyes. It's not just my paranoia. Many despise us. Like a covey of Amish in a casino, we hippies stand out. Our dress, our speech, and our values set us apart. This is the country we were born in, but we are strangers in a strange land.

I don't like Stacy going out alone after dark.

🌟

I let out my air and get on with my work. While he's gone, I'll wash diapers. This is not my favorite chore, but we aren't going to Duluth for another week and it's my turn. I'm in luck. Before he left, my companion hauled two buckets of water up from the river.

First I pour the water in a big tin pan on the cookstove. While it heats, I rinse the soiled nappies in cold. When the water is hot, I scrub them with homemade soap, rinse twice, and two hours later they hang on a rope across the kitchen. Mica is asleep upstairs in his little bed and I stand on the porch, listening for Stacy. He's been gone a long time. Dogs bark in the distance.

"Whoo. Whoo," I yell into the blackness. "Whoo. Whoo."

Stacy has no lantern, and along the trail that stretches between our home and the mailbox there are roots you can trip on, rocks you could crack your head open on, and a treacherous swamp to cross.

"Whoo. Whoo," I call again, but there's only the roar of the river. The quarter moon rises; just a faint glow on the horizon but the Lester reflects the circle of light. A great horned owl, a quarter mile down-river, picks up the call. *Hoo-hoo hoooooo hoo-hoo.* I picture his round eyes piercing the gloom.

Then "Whoooo," very faint. At first when I hear it, I think the owl mocks me, but from faraway in the swamp, Stacy's voice comes again. "Whoo. Whoo."

CHAPTER 2

Peace

"Aren't you worried?" I yell down. "Winter's almost here. Aren't you worried about the cold?"

It's raining again and the roof leaks like a sieve. Every two hours, I empty the containers under the eaves and quickly replace them. Only the west side, where we sleep, is dry. Because of the wind, we can't make repairs.

The swollen Lester River surges past our cabin. We can't get close to the swimming hole or anywhere near the small island where the old pine tree stands. Biting the inside of my lower lip, I watch the raging water from the upstairs window and wonder at what we're doing, trying to live on this eighty-acre subsistence farm, growing our own food, building our dwelling out of recycled materials, living as lightly on the earth as possible. Are we going too far?

Then I clatter down the stairs in my jeans and heavy boots. "Aren't you concerned about the weather, Stacy?"

"Nah, there'll be some good days to work outside yet. There's not much left to do and we'll finish sometime. Think about it. The old couple I met at the end of Dahl Road made it through winter in the old days." Stacy refers to the Olsens, our closest neighbors, the people he visited the night he was away so long.

He mixes another batch of the caulking material and hands me a trowel. Fingers of cold reach into the room and this is still October. *What will it be like by December?* I shake that thought away.

Stacy has his own steady rhythm. He works calmly at one pace, then when up against it, works harder, but I have a sense of urgency and don't like leaving things to the last minute. Slap, I squish on the putty. Whoosh, I smooth the cookie-dough-like substance into the crevice.

7

Paul and Silas bound in jail . . . That's Stacy singing an old freedom song. *Had no money for to go their bail.* Music has always been important to me. I can trace my life story by the soundtrack playing in the back of my mind. *Keep your eyes on the prize, hold on . . .*

All afternoon, we sing as we work. We take turns entertaining the baby and emptying the buckets of water and the rain keeps pounding. My wrists are sore and my arms aching but I'm not stopping until Stacy does.

"Quitting time," Stacy finally announces, picking up Mica and throwing him up to the ceiling. I cringe; the baby's head comes so close to a beam. *Why do men do such things? I can't remember ever seeing a woman toss a baby, certainly not a mother.* Little Mica laughs uproariously and I see why Stacy thinks it's so fun.

In the fading light, my friend washes our tools in the bucket. I warm up our bean soup and muffins and light the lamp. Tonight, as is our custom before eating, we make a circle with our hands, even the baby. As we do, I imagine we're holding hands with all the nonviolent revolutionaries we've known. I look around at the unfinished walls, the piles of clothes, tools, and building supplies, and shake my head. Stacy's probably right. I worry too much.

Warmth from the cookstove, rain on our roof, the three of us safe in our little log cabin. In the glow of the kerosene lamp, Stacy's eyes are moist. I feel the same way. "Peace," Stacy whispers, and we sing our Johnny Appleseed song. *The Lord's been good to me, and so I thank the Lord, for giving me the things I need: the sun and the rain and the apple tree. The Lord's been good to me . . .*

Thou Shalt Not

"Have you heard from Colin?"

Aaron, our friend from Chester Creek House, pulls an extra wooden chair up to the kitchen table. He's a tall guy with dark wild curly hair and a toothy smile that makes you grin even if you aren't in the mood. He showed up this morning saying he was just on a hike, but he must have sensed how desperately we needed him. We've spent all afternoon, under the Minnesota blue sky, nailing down new roofing paper.

Fortunately Mica can sleep through anything and took a long nap while we worked. Forty feet up, as the men walked back and forth on the peaked roof, I crawled on my hands and knees, scared shitless but determined to keep up with them.

"Have you heard from Colin lately?" I repeat.

"He just got out of jail in Hartford after the demonstration at the nuclear submarine base. Bad scene. Fasted without food and water for two weeks." Aaron's mouth tightens and he fiddles with his spoon. I watch his long fingers flip the cutlery back and forth.

"When he was finally taken to court he'd lost twenty pounds. It's only his jailers that kept him alive. They forced water down his throat with a tube every day." The man we speak of is our mutual friend, a full-time activist from the Committee for Non-Violent Action in Connecticut.

Stacy shakes his head. We've all been in jail for a few days, or a few weeks. Some of my draft-resister friends have been incarcerated for years. Stacy, Johan, Aaron, and Colin are only free now because they drew high numbers in the draft lottery. Whether a guy gets a 30 or a 300 can mean the difference between living free and protesting the war, leaving friends and family for Canada, fighting in the jungles of Vietnam, or going to prison as a draft resister.

We all admire Colin's commitment but frown on his extremism, fearing someday he'll die from one of his water fasts . . . or be beaten to death by frustrated guards. I listen as the men discuss the state of the peace movement. Far away from the napalm and death, the war in Vietnam still defines us.

☙

The men's conversation veers to an analysis of Nixon's five-point peace plan and the latest riot at the University of Wisconsin in Madison. A professor was killed in an explosion targeting a research facility aligned with the Defense Department.

"Guys, I'm beat. I'm gonna crash. There's a pile of quilts on the floor by the heater stove or you can sleep with us in the big bed, Aaron." I give him a one-armed hug and lean over to kiss Stacy, who pats me on the butt.

Upstairs, Mica plays with my long loose chestnut hair as he nurses. It saddens me when I hear of Students for a Democratic Society's violent demonstrations. Stacy and I are both against the war for moral reasons, but he has always been more politically sophisticated. My pacifism is simple. I learned it in Sunday school. *Thou shalt not kill.* You can die for the cause and some have, but you don't kill. Pretty simple.

In the window's reflection over the bed, I see my image as an Andrew Wyeth painting, *Farm Woman, Nursing.* I'm not beautiful; in fact as I look at myself I have many complaints, but when I've desired a man, I've usually slept with him. I study my face, unlined, my soft white breasts in the golden lamplight. Colin was the only man who made it clear he wasn't interested. I was in love with him once, maybe still am.

Downstairs the soundtrack to our life starts up again, Stacy on the Autoharp and Aaron on the harmonica. *They're rolling out the guns again, hurroo, hurroo. They're rolling out the guns again . . .* The moonlight streams metallic through the window at the head of the bed, and their song goes up through the rafters, out the patched roof.

But they'll never take our sons again . . . Becoming a mother has changed me; life always seemed precious, but even more so after I gave birth.

No, they never will take our sons again. Johnny I'm swearing to you.

MICA

I look over at Mica lying next to me and touch the little brown birthmark by his right ear. The night I went into labor, I was two weeks past my due date and we'd returned home late from a meeting on alternative lifestyles at the university. I went straight upstairs with an aching back, but had hardly gotten into bed when my water broke. We were living in Duluth, at the Draft Counseling Center, with our friends Ernie and Darla and their three-year-old twins.

"Guess what?" I rolled over and nudged Stacy. "It's started."

We lay holding hands and timed contractions until dawn, then crowded into Ernie's old Chevy and took Route 61 along the north shore to Two Harbors Hospital, the only facility within 150 miles that would let the father be in the delivery room. The sky was turning pink and Lake Superior reflected the sunrise. White seagulls cut the air and I wasn't afraid.

꙾

There's an old wives' tale that if your mother had a fast labor you will, too, but I'm sorry to say, in my case the old wives were off. My mom had me in two hours with hardly a pain, but my baby was sunny-side up, facing the pubic bone instead of the sacrum, a position that causes slow dilatation and constant back pain.

By 10:00 a.m. I was five centimeters, and Stacy joked that I might have the baby by noon. Then progress slowed. The nurses wouldn't let me walk, so I threw off my blue hospital gown and swayed on the bed, on my hands and knees, naked. Shocked, they stopped coming into the room.

Stacy rubbed my lower back for hours and timed the contractions while I did the *hee-hee*'s and *hoo-hoo*'s we'd learned at the Lamaze class in Minneapolis. He was my rock, keeping me centered, suggesting changes of position. Whenever I'd get off track, he'd help me relax.

For hours I stared out the hospital room window across a wide expanse of snow. I saw the light change; the shadows lengthen then turn to dusk. Nothing moved except an occasional car on the road a mile away. I was grateful even for that, any distraction, something to take my mind off the grinding pressure in my sacrum.

There were five pine trees in the field and one of them, if you looked at it right, had a face. The woman I saw there gave me strength. *You can do it!* she would say as I stared at her through contractions. *You can do it. Just take the contractions one at a time.*

By ten at night I had the urge to push and was taken into the delivery room, a green-tiled space dominated by a gleaming silver instrument table and a stainless steel platform with stirrups. I wasn't strapped down like in most hospitals, but I was still flat on my back. Stacy supported my shoulders. If he wasn't touching me, I panicked.

I pushed and I pushed until the veins stood out on my neck like an Amazon warrior and my face turned blue, but nothing moved. Two hours later Dr. Leppink, our peacenik physician, arrived and told the nurses I was pushing too early. I was only eight centimeters. That's when I lost it and took the Demerol.

It wasn't pleasant, but sometimes you just have to choose, medication or insanity, and I'll admit, it relaxed me while we waited for my cervix to withdraw. My disorientation from the medication was worse for Stacy than me. I couldn't keep my eyes open and was incoherent. The combination of no sleep for two days and the drug made me hallucinate. It took another ninety minutes, but finally my cervix was fully dilated.

When at last they took me back to the delivery room, feeling the baby move down spontaneously gave me hope. Getting sugar water in my IV gave me strength. In the end, forceps and a large mediolateral episiotomy were necessary, but it didn't matter.

Birth always alters you. It's a learning experience, and what Stacy and I came to understand is that no matter how many classes you go to, how much you practice relaxation, how many books you read, or how many prayers you put out into the universe, childbirth is beyond your control, a force of nature, like a tornado, a blizzard, or an earthquake.

꙳

As Dr. Leppink pulled and I pushed, the baby shifted.

"Look down," the nurses said. "See your baby being born."

I could feel each part of his body slip out. His head. His shoulders and feet. Then, flop, a wet life on my stomach. This I didn't expect. Babies were usually dangled in midair to drain mucus, spanked, and given to the nurses.

Mica, our son, let out a cry and flung his trembling arms wide. *A baby all wrinkled and tired! Our baby.* Stacy is crying. I am crying. We're exhausted. We're elated.

We made this new being out of our imperfect love; gave life to him from our common belief in a universe that says *yes*.

CHAPTER 3

Shadow

"So, are you up for it?" Stacy looks out the window. "The teach-in isn't for three days, but we could go to town early."

The sun is just rising and, as it warms, the mist lifts off the golden water. A cardinal sits like a drop of blood on the curved cedar tree. I inspect our provisions on the shelves under the kitchen counter, jars that once contained beans, wheat berries, cornmeal, and powdered milk. It's been weeks since we've been to the city or seen anyone but each other. The food containers are mostly empty, but our money jar's empty too.

"Maybe you could get work at the docks. We're low on supplies, plus I want to make some posters for my introductory childbirth class and put them up in the library."

❦

Fine snow blows like sand as we cross the fallen elm that serves as our bridge over the Lester. Stacy, wearing a heavy hooded parka, carries Mica on his back in the baby carrier, first through the woods and then across Jacobsen's pasture to the Jean Duluth Road. We pass shallow pools of marshland surrounded by cattails that harbor mallards and mergansers. They rise as we pass.

"Hi, ducks. Better hurry south. Winter's here." I pull my rainbow scarf tighter, lean into the wind, and review my mental list of what we'll buy in town. Whole-wheat berries to grind into flour, pinto beans and cheese from the natural foods co-op. But we also need nails. Maybe we can borrow some money from Aaron.

Amazingly, as soon as we stick out our thumbs, we're in luck. A beat-up blue pickup pulls over. "It's a cold one," the driver grumbles, leaning over and throwing open the passenger door. I'm assaulted by my childhood smells, cigarettes and beer, but settle myself in the middle of the front seat with Mica in my lap.

"So," says the old guy, dressed in gray coveralls with a green John Deere cap, "what you fellas doing way out here?" I realize that with my braids tucked inside my hood, a wind-burned face, and no makeup, he thinks I'm a man. "Name's Tollefson," he bites out. His face is a wrinkled road map and he has one large dark mole, shaped like Lake Superior, under his eye.

"I'm Stacy Woodrow and this is Patsy, and Mica, our boy." Stacy doesn't call me his wife, but implies it, letting the man know I'm a girl. The driver gives me a quick once-over, adjusting to my femaleness, and pulls back on the road. "Whatcha doing way out here?" he asks again.

"We live about two miles back, on the Lester. Bought eighty acres and built a cabin by the river." I let Stacy do the talking, happy just to be warm and out of the wind. Hitchhiking always makes me wary.

Mica pulls at my coat, wanting to nurse, but embarrassed in such close proximity to Mr. Tollefson, I distract him by playing patty-cake. The radio's tuned to the news and I catch a report that the Khmer Rouge attacked an airport in South Vietnam, but the driver impatiently reaches over and turns the sound off.

"I remember the family that used to own your place, the Lindquists." Tollefson rubs his grizzled white whiskers. "They lost their eighty acres to taxes four years ago. Weren't too happy about the state repossessing it. Farm had been in the family for generations. They had to move into Duluth. That how you got the place? Foreclosure from the county?"

Stacy answers yes, not saying more.

I frown. I'd never thought about who owned our land before, just assumed someone died or maybe flew south, like a migrating bird, to avoid the harsh winters. The thousand dollars we paid for the property was what we had left after Stacy gave his grandmother's inheritance away.

"When the rich die and give their money to their children, they just perpetuate the class system," Stacy had explained to me as he wrote checks to the ACLU, the American Friends Service Committee, and the

War Resisters League. The ethics of inheritance had never occurred to me. In my family, we'd be lucky to get enough for the burial.

Mica falls asleep against my chest. The rough sound of the motor reverberates in the cold. Our driver works his jaw back and forth like a saw and drums on the steering wheel with his weathered hands. I'm not sure if he resents us for buying the Lindquists' farm or just doesn't have anything else to say. Twenty minutes later, we pull up in front of the brick post office in downtown Duluth.

"Thanks, we really appreciate the lift." That's Stacy.

"Yeah, thanks," I chime in.

As we stride down the sidewalk toward Chester Creek House, I glance over my shoulder. Tollefson hasn't moved, and I turn back and wave. The man seems friendly enough. He picked us up when many people wouldn't. But he doesn't wave back.

Chester Creek House

Whitewashed stone walls. A worn red oriental carpet. Mattress on the floor with an Indian-print cotton spread. I'm in our room in the basement of Chester Creek House, folding clean diapers.

The cold light from one tiny window up near the ceiling illuminates Mica, who's playing with wood blocks at my side. On the wall hangs a picture I drew after Mica's birth, showing how I felt after twenty-four hours of constant back labor and three hours of pushing: a wet noodle, but powerful too.

When Mica finally was born, even though the doctor had to help at the end, I felt I could do anything, move a two-ton truck with my bare hands, lift a mountain, part the waters of Lake Superior. In the drawing, which is done in pastels on a large sheet of stiff white paper, Stacy stands guard at the end of the bed, saying, "Push!" On his chest is an H, for My Hero.

It was his strength that got me through the long labor. Women often say they couldn't have done it without their support people. I know now that's true. The pain would suck you down under the earth. People who love you are your anchor to life.

❦

"Shit!" The front door of the three-story Victorian communal house bangs open and male voices echo from the front hall. "My hands are freezing."

It's Stacy, Aaron, and Jim, a pale, quiet, ponytailed refugee from the Kent State massacre, where the Guardsmen fired sixty-seven rounds into the crowd and four students were killed, one paralyzed, and eight others wounded. For three days they've worked unloading cargo ships while I hung around Chester Creek House.

"Hey," I call out, hurrying upstairs with Mica on my hip. "How'd it go?"

The men are pulling off their boots and combing the frost from their beards and mustaches. "We were lucky; another ship came in from the Soviet Union," Stacy tells me. "It might be the last." They're tired and cold, but have cash in their pockets.

Duluth, at the westernmost end of Lake Superior, is linked, via the Great Lakes and the Saint Lawrence Seaway, to the Atlantic Ocean, over twenty-three hundred miles away. Like any seaport, it's a great place to get day labor . . . I'd try it myself, but they don't hire women.

❦

The smell of garlic and cheese fills the house, and it's already dark as we seat ourselves around the long dining table. The Benders, Terry, Joan, and their three kids, have made vegetarian lasagna, tossed salad, and homemade bread for all thirteen of us. Courtney, a pensive, dark-eyed librarian, serves us from the end of the table.

"Patsy and I will split tomorrow. I have fifty-five dollars and we're set for another month, but we want to chip in on the food. We put five bucks in the kitchen money jar," Stacy announces. Though we act like it's not important, money here, as in most communes, is a sensitive issue. As a group, we declare, "To each according to his need and from each according to his ability," but without regular jobs, Stacy and I can't afford to live like the rest of them.

Since last summer, when we gave up our beautiful window-lined bedroom on the second floor and moved down to the basement of this big old Victorian, our role in the community has been awkward. We don't contribute to the rent but still crash at the house when we're in town. Everyone says we're welcome, but I'm concerned their generosity has a limit; that's why I've been helping Leila, Aaron's new girlfriend, paint their turreted bedroom for the last three days . . . to contribute labor instead of cash. Even before we officially moved out, these issues were a tug-of-war.

"Forget it," says Patrick, the balding ex-priest, now a history teacher at Holy Rosary School. "You need the bread more. We'll sponge off *you* sometime."

That's my cue. "We'd be happy to share the farm . . ." I flash him my innocent blue eyes and take another delicate bite of lasagna. For two years, Stacy and I have tried to get these friends to join us on the land. The group laughs uncomfortably and I join in, but my laughter's tinged with resentment and everyone knows this. I catch Stacy's eye. He flashes me a look to cool it.

The fact is that Stacy and I *are* ambivalent about sharing the land. We yearn for community and believe in land trusts, but don't really want to give up control. If these people join us on the farm, even for just the short three-month growing season, they'll bring chain saws, power lines, and vehicles, ripping our Ansel Adams wilderness apart.

Jim pushes his chair back, escaping the rough edges around the table, and slips into the living room, where he turns down the lights and tunes up his twelve-string. One by one, eager to avoid the mealtime strain, we trail after him and slouch on sofa and chairs.

When the sun comes up and the first quail calls, follow the drinking gourd, Jim sings.

For the old man is a waitin' for to carry you to freedom. Follow the drinking gourd, we all join in.

Outside, the wind whips the dark cold. Our relationship with these friends is complicated.

Like yarn, we unravel and then run straight. We have to be careful with each other's feelings, but when we sing, our frayed edges mend.

Left foot, peg foot, travelin' on. Follow the drinking gourd.

From the Heart

Like actors in the musical *Hair,* when Stacy and I stride into the teach-in, friends immediately surround us. "Hey, how you doing?" "We miss you, man." "What's been happening?"

The university auditorium is almost full and I hear a young woman in the audience ask her companion, "Who's that?"

"Stacy and Patsy," the bearded man whispers. "Local war resisters, legendary hippies."

Stacy, wearing jeans and the green tweed sweater I knit him, precedes me to the folding table where the other panelists sit. I follow, tall, confident hippie chick in a long skirt, with her towheaded kid on her back, scanning the packed hall for Johan. I know he's still in Duluth, because Courtney told me he lives with a new girlfriend. I can't find Patrick or Jenny, either; or the Benders and their three kids, the other residents of Chester Creek House. Only Jim is accounted for, leaning against the back wall near the double doors in his patched bell-bottoms and faded denim work shirt. I tilt my chin hello. Aaron said he'd be late.

As the room quiets, Stacy stands and gazes across the waiting faces. Nearly every seat is filled, with college students, activists, and a few professors. A pregnant blond, her long straight hair pulled back with a silver clip, excuses herself, trying to squeeze along the row to an empty place. It's my friend Jody Innis. I smile and wave with my fingers.

Stacy waits and then begins as if we're gathered in someone's living room. "Not since the Civil War has this country been so affected by a military conflict. Every American family is impacted by the war in Southeast Asia. We've lost husbands . . . sons . . . daughters . . . nephews . . . and friends. Who here knows someone who's died in Vietnam?" Hands go up all over the auditorium. "Over forty thousand Americans have been killed already, and many who've returned suffer physical and emotional scars. Nearly *two million* Vietnamese are dead or maimed, destroyed by this war that Nixon promised to end."

When Mica begins to fuss, I throw a knit shawl over him, pull up my turtleneck, and put him to my breast. He nestles against me and I rub

his fine white hair. Stacy addresses the crowd with quiet moral authority, sure of himself and his cause of peace.

The audience is mesmerized. This man has his flaws. He's stubborn.
He procrastinates. He has difficulty compromising and is slightly dys-
lexic, but he speaks eloquently.

When it's my turn, Stacy takes Mica on his shoulders and strolls to
the back of the room to stand with Jim. I tell the audience how the im-
ages on TV tore me from my conventional middle-class life. Vietnamese
monks burning themselves to death to protest the war. Asian mothers
in shock, wandering through the rubble of their homes carrying the
lifeless bodies of their babies . . . I speak from the heart.

From the eyes of the blond with the silver Navaho hair-clip, I know
that at least one person understands.

Intruders

"Stacy!" I point down at the deep boot tracks in the new snow, not un
usual for November in the North Country. We're on our way back to
the homestead after our stay in Duluth, trekking first across Jacobsen's
white field and then through the forest toward the cabin. Dust devils of
powder whirl up in our path.

My companion relishes the subarctic seasons. He thrives on hardship, pointing out the white sculptured drifts, the low purple clouds, and
a red-tailed hawk in an oak tree, while I complain silently. *It's too cold.
I'm too tired. I want to go back to the warmth of Chester Creek House.* "Stacy!"
I hiss again. "Look. Tracks."

My lover bends low, inspecting the human imprint, touching the icy
outline with one finger. "They're fresh and lead toward the cabin. By
the look of the treads, two men." We stand for a moment listening . . .
then with urgency, plow forward, race to the small clearing on the
Lester, another quarter mile away.

At the edge of the open space where our log house sits, Stacy halts,
puts down the baby carrier, and silently hands Mica over to me. He
creeps forward. I hold my breath.

"What the fuck!"

"Stacy?" I flounder up the slope to see my lover positioned on our porch, his stance wide, glaring at the door where the window is shattered. Cautiously we step in and look around, but there are no rocks on the inside, no log or projectile laying there, just a half-inch of snow covering the floor in a wide arc. I picture the intruders using the butt of a gun to smash in the glass. So far from the road, in this clearing in the woods, we thought we'd be safe.

While Stacy builds a fire, I inspect everything; our books, our cooking utensils, our food, our clothing, our tools, our Autoharp and guitar, even Mica's toy box. Nothing seems missing, but I can smell the coarse strangers in our home, tobacco and something else . . . a heavy aftershave. We must have just missed them.

Stacy pounds a square of cardboard over the busted window. Neither of us speaks. The broken window is a warning. A reminder that someone in Lakewood Township doesn't like us; doesn't want us here.

At bedtime, an animal howls far away. "Hear that?" I ask, pulling the thick quilt up to my chin.

"It's just dogs." Stacy blows out the lantern.

"But what's making them bark? *Something's* out there in the dark." I snuggle up to him.

"Just a skunk or a porcupine." In less than two minutes, Stacy's breath deepens. I roll on my back, eyes wide, staring into the shadows as the distant yapping continues. I remember the night the attackers came to the Committee for Non-Violent Action farm, drunken men, in pickups, with guns. That time, too, the dogs barked. Then bullets shattered the window glass.

Here in the woods, we're as vulnerable as isolated settlers squatting on Indian land. If someone were to creep through the woods with intentions to hurt us, there's no way to call for help. We could be dead for two weeks before anyone knew.

Winter

CHAPTER 4

Blizzard

Winter has settled around us for sure. No more bare ground, and little by little the white builds up until we have to use snowshoes.

Last night I woke to the impact of what felt like a bull moose smashing the side of the house, a blast so hard it shook the windows.

"What is it?" I ask Stacy, sitting up in bed.

"Just the wind."

All night it howls. In the morning eight inches of new snow loads the balsam grove, and while Stacy is out cutting firewood, four more inches fall. I look out the window, angry at the weather. We'd planned to go into town for my childbirth class at the library, but there's no way with this storm and this grieves me.

Up until now there have been no natural-childbirth classes north of the Twin Cities. No hospital where a woman can have natural childbirth with the father present, until we convinced Dr. Leppink, in Two Harbors, to let us give it a try.

Stacy and I took the four-hour Greyhound bus trip eight times in eight weeks to go to Lamaze classes in Minneapolis. It was a big sacrifice, but both of us were working then, so we had the bread.

That's why I've tried to start the childbirth class at the library; so expectant parents wouldn't have to go so far. I have no more qualifications than having taken the course myself, read several books, and, of course, given birth; how can I gain credibility if I don't show up? I know of at least four couples that were planning to come. There probably were more. Hopefully someone will realize why I'm not there.

※

The wind rages all day, battering the cabin, hard gusts against the house, with flakes so thick you can't see the maple tree where the red squirrel

22

lives. Snow like a white curtain drops over our world. I take notice of our diminishing provisions. Already the jars of pinto beans, cornmeal, and oats are near empty. *If the snow gets too deep, how long can we last?* My stomach feels hollow when I remember how cut off we are.

Life, I suppose, goes on as usual in Duluth. Leila and Courtney are baking bread at Chester Creek House while the Bender kids chase each other around the dining table. Aaron and Jim are attending the War Resisters meeting in a crowded classroom at the university. Afterward they'll join Johan to prepare the next issue of our alternative newspaper, *The Wild Currents,* while Stacy and I are trapped in the middle of a snow globe.

※

The blizzard lasts for three days. We read. We play with Mica in the dim kerosene lamplight. We make love while the baby naps. We go to bed early to conserve fuel. There's nothing to do but hibernate like bears, keep warm, and wait. Leaving the cabin is too dangerous. A body could get lost in the blanket of white, get confused and wander off through the forest.

On the third day, just before dawn, the howling stops. I wake, startled by silence, scoot to the window at the end of the bed, and scrape off the frost. At the top of the curved cedar that hangs over the Lester, I see stars when the clouds part. "It's over," I whisper to Stacy. "It's over."

※

Morning. Sunny and blue. I stand Mica up on the window seat and let him peek out while I pull on his blue nylon snowsuit. In the clearing, Stacy and I throw our arms wide, demonstrate how to make snow angels, and laugh when we fall back, the white stuff so fluffy and deep it covers us. We're playing like kids when we hear a crack in the underbrush and go on alert. I hold our little boy protectively.

Gunshots

Two men on horseback with four big dogs come out of the trees. They work their horses closer. Mica snuggles into my neck. "Doggie!" he laughs. It's Rob Bailey, our Vietnam vet neighbor, and his brother Ed, dressed like heroes in an old western, their Stetsons pulled low and their wool plaid scarves, like masks, tied over their faces. Since the broken window we've been on edge. Stacy knows Rob from the whole-food co-op. He enjoys discussing the war with him, getting a new perspective. Rob hates Nixon, but thinks peaceniks are sissies. Stacy told him about Vietnam Veterans Against the War and little by little he's coming around.

Rob looks down from his perch on his mount and clears his throat. "You couldn't turn us on to a cup of hot coffee, could you?" The men tie their horses to trees and we tromp inside, pull off our icy boots and jackets, and draw up chairs to the cookstove.

"No coffee," I tell the men. "Too expensive, but this peppermint tea will warm you up."

Ed, a graduate student in biology, leans forward, elbows on his knees. He wears heavy horn-rimmed glasses and, unlike his older veteran brother, who works at the post office, has a full head of yellow hair.

Rob clears his throat and turns toward Stacy; *not wanting to worry the little woman,* I think. "Have you folks heard any gunshots lately?"

Stacy rises and stokes the fire. He steps over Rob's long legs. "Shots?"

"A few nights ago. We weren't sure at first, thought it was maybe backfire from someone's truck, but it was too regular and too close." He picks at the hole in the toe of his sock. "This was the night before the blizzard. We brought in the dogs and checked the horses, but the gunshots went on maybe an hour. The night was pitch-black and colder than hell."

"We called into the dark, but no one answered," Ed cuts in. "After a while the shots just stopped and we went back to bed."

Stacy changes the subject. "How are the roads into town? Pretty bad?" He's unwilling to entertain paranoia.

"Fear of each other just makes things worse," he later tells me, but I'm still thinking of gunshots.

Winter Solstice

"Where shall we have the bonfire?" I ask. It's December 21, the longest night of the year.

The blizzard, three weeks ago, brought it home to us. Winter really is here, and we've worked hard for days finishing the chinking. The little cabin in the woods is now cozy and warm. We've even made Styrofoam plugs that we put in the windows for insulation at night. Laura and Mary in their *Little House in the Big Woods* never had it so good.

Exhausted from cutting and stacking wood all morning, Stacy stares out the kitchen window at the azure sky. A flicker with its white tail and red head pecking high in the maple catches my eye. "Look, Mica. A woodpecker."

"Let's build the fire out in the big clearing." Stacy brushes a few crumbs from his beard. I reach over and pick one off that he's missed.

"At the end, by the rutabaga patch?"

Our first vegetable garden, two summers ago when Mica was only four months old and we lived in a tent, was a poor one. Like yeomen farmers of old, we turned over the sod by hand and dumped in wood ashes, but the soil was still too acid.

Our second garden, this summer, though not great, was an improvement, and what we lost in an abundant harvest we made up for in style. Our whimsical plot was hand-tilled in the shape of a man with his thumb up, hitchhiking. It was Stacy's idea. He's clever like that. You could only appreciate it from an airplane or the top of a pine, but the head was a spiral of thyme, sweet marjoram, and basil. The arm and the thumb were sunflowers.

My lover inspects the angle of the light through the window. "We better build the fire. It'll be dark in an hour."

"There's the brush that we cut at the edge of the clearing." I say this over my shoulder while rinsing my fingers in the washbowl. The sink with no faucets, which we found at the county dump, drains into a slop bucket. Before bed we'll empty it outside in the balsam grove.

※

The three of us bundle up with knit caps, mittens, and scarves over our faces. Mica wears his little blue snowsuit and lined boots, new, from the Goodwill. Out in the clearing, we tramp the snow down for our ceremonial fire and drag a log over to sit on. Though the cold and snow have clamped around us for weeks, today is the first official day of winter.

The fire is roaring as the sun inches behind the pale poplars, sentries at the edge of the woods. I nurse Mica, an old quilt wrapped around us. Now and then he pulls back from the breast, looks up, and says, "'Bye, Sun.'"

All is perfect and still. No sound. No movement, just the clean white snow and the smell of the evergreens. Spires of gold shoot up from the horizon as the last flash of light from the west dies away. The three of us take off our mittens and solemnly raise our palms to the sun, paying tribute to the giver of life on this shortest day of the year, this longest night.

"Ohm," Stacy chants. "Ohm . . ." from deep in his chest. I join him and reach for his work-callused hand. Mica imitates us in his little-boy voice. "Ohm. Ohm." *Peace.*

※

Now our baby crawls all over me, restless as a spider monkey. The moment has passed . . . We take turns kicking snow over the last of the blaze, more for fun, to see the steam rise, than safety, then tromp back through the woods to the cabin. Inside, I put on a kettle for tea and check the firebox. I'm remembering last solstice at Chester Creek House, how we introduced our candle ceremony to the commune. I miss our friends.

"What's that?" Stacy cocks his head. We run to the window. Voices waft through the night. Voices singing. *Over the river and through the woods, to the little log cabin we go!*

The door swings open and Aaron bursts through. "Surprise!" He tosses his cowboy hat on the window seat and shrugs off his parka.

Jim follows, stepping out of his boots. As usual he doesn't say much, just takes a seat at the table, nods hello, and picks up my guitar.

Leila rests her walking stick just inside the door and hangs up her long black wool cape. She gives me a one-armed hug, clips back her ebony hair, and starts pulling goodies out of her knapsack. I am so grateful to these comrades for *remembering* and for tramping all the way through the snowy woods, in the cold and dark, just to join us for solstice.

"Brrrrrr. Give me warmth. It's going to be forty below zero tonight," Aaron says as he drops his cowboy hat over Mica's face. "How you doin', partner?"

Forty below! I observe the stout timber walls and our pile of wood near the stove. A rush of excitement runs through me, as if meeting a cunning opponent. *The cold will not get us tonight. Not if I can help it!*

Stacy encourages everyone to draw up to the table. "Come on. Let's get started." He knows I take this ritual as seriously as if it were Mass, Passover, and Communion rolled into one.

After a moment of silence, we begin to light the assorted candles that I bought at the Salvation Army store. Some are new, some half-gone. "I'll light the red one for fire," Stacy says. We think about that for a minute, on this below-zero night.

"Hot!" Mica announces. *Hot* was one of his first words. In a cabin with a woodstove and kerosene lamps, we've said *hot* to him so often and with such intensity, he picked it up early.

"This blue one is for water," Aaron says, leaning in.

"This tall gold one is for the earth and all that sustains us," Leila whispers. She pulls her hair back as she bends over the flames.

I take my turn. "The white one is for family." I look at Mica, then at Stacy and around at the larger group. They are my family too. Fleetingly I flash on my mother, sitting home alone, watching TV in the living room of our house in Carson City, and my brother, Darren, so far away I don't even know where he lives.

Jim follows, but he takes a long time. "The orange candle is for peace and justice and for those who have died for it . . ." I picture the students at Kent State.

Mica stands up in his highchair, supported by Stacy. "Hot!" he squeals again. All night the candles will burn in their little tin plates until the sun, giver of life and warmth, returns.

When we are done, Aaron leans back and pulls his Hohner harmonica out of his shirt pocket. Stacy opens his Autoharp case and Jim picks up the guitar again. *'Tis a gift to be simple, 'tis a gift to be free* . . . Leila swings me around in an improvised jig. *'Tis a gift to come down where we ought to be* . . . If the stout log walls could dance, they'd pick up and join us.

CHAPTER 5

Tree Song

Christmas comes and goes without much celebrating. Stacy considers it *overcommercialized capitalist crap,* and I sing carols to the trees and the woodland critters down by the river. The days pass with inside work, reading, and playing. The leaden gray sky presses down on us. Tonight while Stacy is out cracking the ice at the spring, I hear him call.

"Patsy! *Paaatsy!*"

Running to the door, I poke my head into the arctic world and gasp as the glacial air greets me. "What?" I shout back. It's pitch black outside, no moon tonight and colder than hell. We've lost our thermometer under the snow, so I don't know *how* cold, just colder than hell.

"Come out here. Get Mica. Come now."

"This better be good," I say under my breath as I bundle us up, tie my rainbow scarf over my lower face, and check Mica's scarf too.

"Listen," Stacy whispers when we reach him, standing with his buckets next to the spring. "Listen . . . ."

I wait, balancing Mica on my hip and staring at my baby with big, expectant eyes. Mica imitates me, giving the same exaggerated round blue eyes back.

Then I hear it, *Ping.* In another few seconds, *Pung.* In five or ten more . . . *Peng. Pong.* Then *Ping* again, like notes on a distant marimba. Every few seconds from near or far, *Ping. Pong. Pung.* Soft or loud, high pitched or low, from ten feet away or down by the river, the forest is making slow music.

"What is it?" I whisper.

Stacy shakes his head and shrugs. "The trees are singing."

"No, *really.*"

"It's the sound of the sap freezing and breaking in the bark, that's my guess. Maybe the reason we never heard it before is, we never stood out in the woods when it was thirty below."

"It's a hymn!"

Ping . . . Pong . . . Pung . . . Ping . . . Peng . . . Pong. There's nothing but pure white untrampled snow and the smell of the balsam and fir. We lean against each other listening to the woodland concert until we're too cold and we must go back inside.

Malcontent

One day fades into the next. White clouds in rows like fish scales. This morning, I take Mica for a ride on a toboggan that I've rigged with a wooden box. He laughs, stretching his red-mittens hands straight out, his white-blond head falling back as he bumps. Later we plant sticks in the snow and call them flowers. Mica is my little pal. When we lie by the river in the sunshine on a leftover piece of Styrofoam, next to the curved cedar, there's no sound but water gurgling under the ice.

Such a simple, decent life, yet something is missing, and often these days I've been frustrated, worrying over our lack of progress, getting upset because nothing ever gets finished. I find myself thinking about people in town, wondering how they are doing. I work on the series of childbirth classes that I've been trying to start but now probably won't.

Our house is warm and tight now, but it's still a dump, and Stacy isn't concerned. His mind is on higher things, nonviolent revolution, saving the planet, stopping the war. Who can find blame?

I try to console myself. *What does it matter about the cabin? Take it easy. You have a roof over your head. You're warm. You have a wonderful family, a bed, a place to cook and play. There are plenty who don't.* My pep talk only works until I can't locate the toilet paper or a book on childbirth I've laid aside; then I'm just pissed. It all feels so futile.

CHAPTER 6

Break in the Weather

"Anyone home?"

It's a brilliant day and I stand at the door, screening my eyes from the snow's intense glare. Jody Innis picks her way down the path, pink, radiant, and very pregnant. "What's happening, little boy?" She grabs Mica, laughs, and throws her long blond braid back over her shoulder.

This is our first human contact, apart from each other, since we went into Duluth for provisions in early February. Mica's as excited as I am but Stacy will miss the visit. He's packed a lunch and gone to cut wood on the other side of the river.

Jody, tall and fair, a Scandinavian goddess, has been my friend since we moved to Duluth. We came across each other at a women's meeting at the university. I sat next to her on the hardwood floor, and when I noticed she laughed at the same things I did, I knew we'd be pals.

"It's so good to see you! Tell me everything," I demand over raspberry tea. "Have you decided which hospital you're going to? Did you call Dr. Leppink, the family doc in Two Harbors? He's the best."

I recall Stacy's and my decision to have our baby in the hospital. We wanted to deliver at home, but there was no midwife. After much research and serious discussion, we chose tiny Two Harbors Hospital, thirty miles north, the only hospital where Stacy was allowed in the delivery room.

There are two larger, better-equipped hospitals in Duluth with OB specialists, but neither institution allows natural childbirth or the father to be present during labor. At both St. Luke's and St. Mary's every woman gets a spinal or gas, whether she needs it or not. Her hands will be strapped to the delivery table and her legs tied open in stirrups. When the infant is delivered, always with forceps over a large vaginal incision, it will be spanked and whisked to the nursery. No gentle

31

natural deliveries. No holding the baby. No nursing immediately after birth. No father present. *Nonnegotiable.*

"Yeah, I called Leppink's office," Jody responds. "They want three hundred dollars up front for the delivery. That's just the doctor's part. It's another three hundred for the hospital stay, and they asked where I'd gotten my prenatal care." I had forgotten how much it costs. Stacy and I were working then and paid a little each week.

"You've been going to the Health Department in Duluth, right?" It's been months since I've seen my friend, not since the fall teach-in. "You went there a few times anyway."

Jody doesn't answer but reaches down for Mica and lifts him up to her lap, or what's left of her lap, now mostly round belly.

"You never went?"

Her hazel eyes dart away like trout in the clear Lester River. "I went to the clinic one time, but I didn't like the nurses. Their faces are hard and they asked me to fill out a form saying who the father was . . . so I left."

"Listen, not getting prenatal care is messed up. So what if they give you a hard time? At least they can tell if the baby's growing and if it's healthy. They'll give you free prenatal vitamins and pamphlets to read."

Jody pats her protruding abdomen. "My baby's growing just fine. Frog got vitamins at the whole-food co-op . . . and I read some library books." She changes the subject. "The cabin looks great. I haven't been here since you put in the windows and shelves. It's so cozy."

I glance around the room at our handiwork. We *have* made some progress. The cupboards are up. There's a fold-down desk in the corner, a painted toy box, even new quilted cushions on the window seat.

"Don't try to distract me. *Who* are you going to get to deliver the baby? And where?"

Jody, like most of us, is a college dropout but she isn't dumb.

"Everything's gonna be fine. Women have been having babies for millions of years. All you have to do is listen to your body." She's winging it here, I can tell. She has no clue of the intensity of the experience that is before her. Frog, her boyfriend, an artist who spends most of his day stoned in front of the woodstove, isn't any better. They live out on Zimmerman Road in an insulated shack that's both his studio and home. Frog lets Jody use his beat-up Ford pickup whenever she needs to go somewhere.

I pour each of us another cup of wild raspberry tea, made from leaves we collected at the edge of the clearing, then get out cornbread and peanut butter. "You want me to go over the childbirth breathing?"

Jody shrugs. "Sure . . . I was thinking maybe you could be my coach. Frog's not much into it."

All afternoon we practice the *hee-hee* and *hoo-hoo* that Stacy and I learned in Lamaze class in Minneapolis. That's why I put up the signs at the library and am trying to get the classes started. Few others would have the money or the will to go to such lengths.

Near dusk, Jody leaves us, waving good-bye as she heads up the trail. The pregnant Madonna worries me. It's one thing to be brave about childbirth. Every woman needs to be brave; it's another thing to be foolhardy.

Invitation

"Well, come on in!" Ila hollers from the kitchen as Barney opens the glass storm door. Inside, the house is dark, with three high, small windows curtained in yellowed lace. There's the smell of old things, like a grandma's house, and something fragrant from the kitchen. On every surface rests some sort of knickknack.

Barney and Ila Olsen, our closest neighbors, the couple Stacy met that dark night he stayed away from the cabin so long, have invited us for Sunday lunch. Mica toddles over to the ceramic owls and lambs, shepherdesses and clowns. "Do you like my pretties?" Ila asks. She's a small, round woman in her late seventies, with thin white hair pinned under a hairnet and very pale blue eyes.

Barney pulls his heavy body up from a worn easy chair and puts the more breakable trinkets on high shelves. You can tell his back hurts him. He's a big man with a reddened farmer's face and a three-day growth of white whiskers. "No-no," he tells Mica. His dark eyes are hard but his voice is gentle.

"Come on to dinner now," Ila calls from the kitchen. Except for Jody, these are the first people we've seen for weeks. We thought when we moved to the land that we would make friends with the locals, that they would become our community, but with six months of winter, our transportation difficulties, and our workload on the homestead, socializing is difficult.

At a sunny table covered with a blue-checkered cloth, we take chairs, waiting, unsure if the couple will say grace. I put Mica's hands in his lap. Sure enough, Barney bows his head and mumbles, "Lord bless this food that Thou has bestowed . . ." I don't catch the rest, he says it so fast.

"Do you like Swedish meatballs?" Ila asks, reaching across the table with a ladle. I meet Stacy's eyes. We'd talked about whether we'd stick to our vegetarian principles, and decided to be polite and eat whatever was served unless there were eyeballs actually staring at us. Swedish meatballs hardly seem like real meat.

"Sure," Stacy responds. "Love 'em." I say a silent *thank you* to the cow that gave us his life, and dig in.

Ila's upper arms jiggle as she plies us with food. Besides the main course, we have a feast of Wonder Bread with real butter, green beans with bacon, mashed potatoes, and, for dessert, red Jell-O, which Mica can't get enough of. This is not our usual organic whole-food diet, but it's delicious and I have second helpings of everything, hoping I don't seem too greedy.

Barney and Ila never had children. They live as isolated as we do. We linger all afternoon in their three-room cottage, chewing the fat. I'm careful not to get into anything political, not wanting to alienate our new friends, but Stacy plows ahead. Turns out, Barney agrees with us about Vietnam. Thinks the whole civil war is none of our damn business.

"We saw some strange tracks back in the woods the other day," Stacy announces. Barney's head goes up.

"Tracks, ya say?"

"Yeah, big ones. Huge!"

I jump in. "We followed them along the river, winding in and out of the swamp, but a storm was coming and we had to get home. Big ones like this." I demonstrate with both hands curved and wide. "With claws!" I was a theater major before dropping out of San Francisco State University.

The old man catches Ila's eye.

"We couldn't decide what they were," Stacy continues mildly. "You have a guess? I figure it was one of Rob Bailey's big dogs."

"Could be, but you better not go down there no more; stay close to your cabin."

I squint. "You think it's *bear?*"

"Could be."

"But it's too early for that. They'd be hibernating, right?"

Barney tips his head sideways and scratches his bristled cheek. "Could still be sleeping, but they might not. We've had some warm days . . ."

I glance at the golden light coming in through the window and realize it's nearly four. The winter days are short in the North and I'm not in the mood to meet a large, hairy, flesh-eating animal out after dark. "I guess we've better get going. The supper was wonderful, Ila. You're a great cook." The old lady giggles and looks at her man.

"She oughta be good. She's had plenty of practice feeding me these last fifty-two years." Barney pats his round belly and stands to help Stacy get Mica into his carrier. "You all need any help over there this spring, give me a holler. I got me a newfangled rototiller."

Hiking home in the gloom, I listen for sounds of a large prowling beast as we pass through the deepest part of the swamp. My stalwart companion warbles to Mica. *This old man, he played one. He played knick-knack on my thumb . . .*

"Stacy," I whisper. "You think there really could be bears?"

Spring

CHAPTER 7

Teacher

"So here's the deal," I tell everyone sitting on the floor and sofas of the community room at the library. "There's nothing magical about childbirth breathing. It just keeps you calm and gives you something to do when you want to run away, which you can't, so you might as well settle down and do your job." The expectant mothers look nervous but the fathers laugh at my little joke.

With Courtney's help, because she works as one of the librarians, I'm finally back on track with my classes. I managed, after the big blizzard, to call her from Rob's trailer out on Dahl Road. She reassured me that she'd covered for me, had the names of the people who showed up, and offered to call them and put up new signs.

"I won't kid you. Contractions hurt. If yours don't, let me know!" This time everyone laughs. Some childbirth teachers don't mention pain, they call it "pressure" or "discomfort," but I want the couples to have a realistic understanding of what they're in for.

Most of these women are now close to term, and I admire them for trying to get all the information they can before the biggest adventure of their lives. Three couples are planning to go to St. Mary's and three to Two Harbors Hospital. One single mom hasn't made up her mind. My heart goes out to her and I'd like to be her coach, but I have no phone and no way to travel from the homestead if she goes into labor at night.

"Can you go over the pushing part one more time?" a bearded guy with a leather headband asks. His wife, a pale blond, cuddles between his legs. "What exactly *is* the guy supposed to do?"

I go over the positions for pushing, how the mother should be as upright as possible. I tell them about back labor. "Get on your hands and knees if that feels better. You can sit straight up or you can see if the nurses will let you squat in the bed before you go into the delivery room. The nurses at Two Harbors just leave you alone if you take off your hospital gown." The pale blond turns red and I realize I've probably gone too far.

"They don't know anything about natural childbirth, but they won't interfere. I wish now that I'd tried squatting. I might not have had to have forceps . . .

"Another tip: try to stay home as long as you can."

Fever

"Shit, I got to throw up again! Can you get me the bowl?"

Stacy pukes and I hand him a washcloth. I feel like Clara Barton, Civil War nurse. Outside, night is falling; the first star already shows, low in the sky.

Mica coughs over and over; his cheeks are flushed. Stacy vomits again but it's only green bile. Both of them have fever and diarrhea, and I can't say I feel so great myself, but I still have to do evening chores. There's no one but me.

Though it's officially spring, there's still a foot of snow on the ground. I bundle up, strap on snowshoes, and waddle like a duck out to the woodpile. The wind almost takes my breath away.

♃

"Do you think we should try to get into the city?" I ask, lying down beside Stacy when I come back inside. He's as hot as the cookstove. "Mica's not getting any better, and he's had a fever for two days. I'm worried. If we could get to Rob Bailey's house early in the morning, we could catch a ride to Duluth. I could carry Mica if you could walk on your own." I stare at my companion's exhausted pale face, his matted hair.

"I might be better by tomorrow."

"Yeah, but you might not. One more day of this and you could be so weak I won't be able to get you out. My bowels are starting to cramp, too, and my chest feels heavy." I stand in an effort to strengthen my argument.

My lover, a Taurus, is a stubborn man. He doesn't change course easily, so I press on. "If *I* get sick, we're really in trouble. Who'll bring in the wood? Who'll keep the fire going and get water? Mica's dehydrated. We've got to get him to a doctor."

Stacy lifts himself up on his elbow, studying our son, who sleeps with one limp hand dangling out of the covers. "A hundred years ago, and in third world countries even today, there would *be* no doctor. The body can heal without medicine."

I close my eyes, take a deep breath, and try again. "Are you hearing me? He's not drinking or nursing. I've experimented with everything. Water, peppermint tea . . ." Our eyes meet. At last Stacy gets it. This is serious; we have to get out.

"Get me some honey and tea. Even if I vomit most of it up, it might give me strength." Stacy pulls up to test himself but falls back on the bed. He's so feeble he can hardly stand upright to pee. Like a tree rotted at the base, he wavers when I hold out the potty.

Before bed, I check the heater stove again and break up some kindling. Mica keeps throwing his covers off. Stacy moans in his sleep. A watchwoman guarding the flame, I sit on the side of the bed until my head drops. I'm all that protects my family tonight from the deep arctic cold.

Forced March

"Stay right behind me," I order as I pull the baby carrier over my shoulders and open the door. "Call if I'm going too fast or you fall." I hand Stacy the walking stick that Leila left last solstice, a stout oak pole, and then I strap on his snowshoes. He's still so feeble I had to dress him. Mica's as hot as a firecracker.

In the night, three inches of new snow has drifted in swirls over the trail and the going is rough, so I break out in song to cheer us. *We are marching to Pretoria, Pretoria . . . Pretoria . . .* My voice rings through the frigid air. *March with me. I'll March with you.* Who do I think I'm kidding? My grandmother might have lived like this as a pioneer in Ontario, but I'm not cut out for it.

I stomp along on our secondhand snowshoes, my chest tearing with each raspy breath, and turn to let Stacy catch up. He plods with his head down, gazing numbly at my tracks. In the swamp where the trail dips into the gulley, we startle four quail out of the snow. They fly up in our faces and make Mica cry. Twice I fall and pick myself up. The ice gets into my mittens.

While I'm down, I notice what a beautiful morning it is. The air is so still and the half moon tilts, silver, in the pale blue sky. Two pink clouds hover on the edge of the sunrise.

The last time I tumble, I twist my snowshoes and drop off the packed path into powder. I'm floundering around, trying to get my footing, one snowshoe twisted behind the other, when Stacy leans over and reaches out for me. "We've got to keep moving," he states, more like his old stalwart self. "If we miss Rob out on Dahl Road, I'm not sure how we'll make it to town. It's too cold to hitchhike."

Yellow light creeps up the birch trees as we hit the end of the plowed road. There's no light in Barney and Ila's house, no smoke from the chimney, and I remember they said they were going to her sister's in St. Paul. A mile farther and we're standing in front of Rob's faded blue trailer, just in time. He's already warming up the truck, and white smoke billows out of the tailpipe.

Forty minutes later, we're tottering unsteadily up the shoveled cement walk toward Chester Creek House. Patrick spies us out the front bowed window and he and Aaron rush to the door. The smell of coffee and whole-wheat toast washes over us and we collapse into the loving arms of our friends.

Leila and Courtney pull off our stiff coats, put palms on our foreheads as mothers do, rub our cold hands between theirs. Jimmy takes Mica out of his carrier. "Shit! This baby is burning up," he observes. "This kid is sick!"

Holy Water

Home again, Stacy and I, dressed in our long johns, are doing yoga before breakfast, stretching up to the high-peaked ceiling, then down to our toes, then way back again, like a bow, saluting the sun. We delight in feeling our bodies strong after a week of rest at Chester Creek House. Eventually I, too, succumbed to the fever and then recovered. I never before understood how people could die of influenza. Now I know. The three of us alone out here in the woods, it could happen.

"Hellooo!" comes a male voice from the clearing. "Helloooooo!" with an edge of desperation. "Anyone there?"

We quickly pull on our jeans and sweatshirts and bounce down the stairs to find Frog, Jody's partner, at the door. As soon as he comes into the cabin, his wire-rim glasses steam from the warmth and he lays them on the wooden kitchen counter before he speaks. "Jody told me I should come for you. It's started."

I begin to gather my things, my rainbow scarf and boots and a tattered paperback copy of *Childbirth without Fear*. I wasn't expecting Jody to go into labor so soon. A quick mental calculation and I realize that she's thirty-eight weeks. At the door, I kiss Stacy. Then Mica. Our one-year-old is still nursing, but he gets most of his nutrition from table food.

"See you tomorrow," I say optimistically. "Mama's got to go help Frog and Jody get a baby." I give Stacy another distracted kiss on the side of his cheek. He grabs my hand and squeezes.

I'm looking forward to participating in a birth. The only one I've seen so far was my own, in a mirror.

With this break in winter's grip, water is everywhere. It wets the dark trunks of the maples and oaks. It drips from the tips of the fir needles and the blackberry bushes. It bubbles through the swamp where we cross the creek. Frog and I slog back along the thawing trail without talking.

Thirty minutes later we're in his old truck. The sky's dotted with horsetail clouds from horizon to horizon, and the half-frozen road is slick with mud. I try to make small talk.

"How's Jody doing?" I shout over the roar of the motor.

"Don't know. Been gone almost two hours wandering around in the woods looking for you." He says this like I was purposely hiding.

For three miles there's more silence, and I take the opportunity to observe my driver. Frog's high cheekbones and thin nose speak of aristocratic ancestors. I think of rich landlords in Spain or Italy. His gentle mouth curves over his straight white teeth, but he doesn't smile. No beard, but a five o'clock shadow.

We bounce down Zimmerman, another gravel road, to his two-room wooden shack. Smoke drifts out of the tin stovepipe, but the front windows are still covered with frost. Frog pulls into the side drive and leaves the truck running.

"You go on in, I've got to make a run to Aesop's farm out on Lavis for some milk and eggs."

"*Now?* You won't be gone long will you? What if it's time to go to the hospital?"

"I'll just be away a few minutes." *You'd think he'd want to check on Jody's progress before he left.*

When I enter, the enclosed wooden front porch is chilly and smells of cedar. Jackets, snowshoes, and hats of all kinds hang on the inner wall, and split wood is stacked up everywhere. A black lab leaps up to greet me.

"Jody?"

On the other side of the wall, Bob Dylan sings on the stereo in his reedy voice. Something about a girl from the North Country. *Fitting,* I think. The inner door flies back, almost hitting me.

"Sorry," Jody laughs. "Were you standing there long? I was just building up the fire . . . Where's Frog?" She stuffs the piece of cedar into the heater stove, then pushes down on her knees to hoist her heavy body erect. From her good cheer I deduce she's not in hard labor.

"He said he had to make a run for milk and eggs to some farm out on Lavis Road. You doin' OK?" The tall, pregnant woman is dressed in a blue calico skirt that comes down to her ankles, and a green turtleneck sweater. Her straight blond hair is twisted up on her head.

I can't help comparing us. I wear jeans, heavy work boots, and a red flannel shirt with my hair in two braids, a good-looking, healthy peasant farmwoman, but Jody is regal, a match for Lord Frog. I could be her maidservant, she the lady of the manor; only, this wooden bungalow is hardly a castle.

I take in the room. A chaotic collection of impressionist oil paintings depicting bleak northern landscapes covers the whitewashed wooden walls. Worn oriental carpets are spread on the floor. An easel sits in the corner. "Did Frog paint these? He's very talented."

Jody raises one eyebrow. "Talented yes, when he works, but it's not milk he's going after. It's pot. He's almost out. And yeah, I'm fine. A little tired." *So much for husband-coached childbirth.*

The mother-to-be stops, tilts her head, and stares into space. "Here comes one now." I pick up an old wristwatch with one leather band that rests on top of *The Emergency Childbirth Manual* and place my hand on Jody's belly. The mild pain lasts thirty seconds, and a long day stretches before us. "You slept last night, didn't you?"

"Not much. After my water broke, I was too excited, but I finally drifted off for a few hours this morning."

"Your water broke? Frog didn't tell me. Did you ever get to the Health Department?" Jody shakes her head no and, smoothing her skirt, avoids my eyes. "I couldn't get in. They only do prenatal visits on Friday, and Frog had the truck."

"Did you at least call the doctor . . . ?" I'm interrupted by the sound of a motor in the drive and the slam of the truck door. Frog comes in whistling.

"How's it going, ladies?" He gives Jody a kiss, all jolly now. *It must be good dope.* Jody twists away. Then she gets that faraway look in her eye again and starts rubbing her abdomen.

"Six minutes apart that time," I announce. I wait, and watch, as the square of sunlight from the six-paned window creeps across the floor. Frog makes us raspberry tea. He offers me a joint, but I decline.

"You got around to calling Dr. Leppink, didn't you, Jody?" No answer. "Jody?"

Frog picks up his guitar and croons in a reedy tenor. *Take this road to the dawn's early light . . .*

"I tried, but they were already closed and then I forgot. I don't want to go to the hospital." Another contraction and I realize the pains are coming four minutes apart now. This is crazy . . . The woman has had no prenatal care and no doctor or midwife lined up for the delivery. *How did I get involved in this mess?*

Another contraction and Jody's eyes get big. "Mmmmph. That one was hard."

"Jody?" I touch her face. "What do you mean you don't want to go to the hospital? This is nuts. Your water's been broken for almost twenty hours and we don't even know if the baby's head-down. If it's breech we're in trouble." Jody moans again. "Do you understand what I'm saying?"

"I don't want to go. We can do it here. You'll help me."

I stare around the room as if the walls and the paintings could give me some help.

"Maybe we can stay here for a little while longer, but I'm telling you, I'm *not* delivering this baby, and neither is Frog."

Jody bends low and groans. "Here comes more fluid." She holds her skirt up between her legs like a woman stomping grapes.

"Towels!" I order Frog, who gets to his feet and saunters into a back room.

For the next two hours, Jody paces, Frog strums his guitar, and I worry. Time halts during contractions and then starts up again. Around five, I notice perspiration on Jody's top lip and she won't talk to me anymore. She sways back and forth, her eyes closed.

"Jody, I really think your labor is progressing. Do you have gloves, like exam gloves? Maybe I should try to check you."

"I was gonna get some at the drugstore next week. I have alcohol though. You could wash your hands in that."

"Yeah, I got some booze," adds Frog with a grin, and I give him a look. *Seventh-grader.*

"OK, where's the rubbing alcohol? I'll wash my hands in it and make sure the head's coming, but I'm telling you again we have to get out of here in the next hour or so." Jody bends low and groans. I'm remembering my friends Joshua and Sunny, who tried to deliver their own infant at home on Tolstoy Farm in Washington. This was after we left the West Coast for the Committee for Non-Violent Action farm in Connecticut, where we lived with Colin. The baby was breech and he died.

I have imagined so many times the parents' horror, seeing little blue feet coming out when they expected a head, hearing silence instead of the newborn's first cry, holding a cold, gray baby without a heartbeat instead of a warm, pink one.

"Here comes more water." Jody holds her skirt up again.

"More towels!" I order Frog, who gets to his feet and again shuffles into the back room.

"Jody, come over here and lie down. I'm going to check you." I pat the bed. "If the baby is headfirst and you aren't much dilated, we can stay here another few hours. Where's the alcohol?"

"Dresser!" Jody barks.

I wait until she's done with her next contraction, then stand over the sink and pour the clear, cold liquid on my two longest fingers. Jody spreads her legs.

I have no clue what I'm feeling for. *What makes me think I can find her cervix?* Then I feel resistance, something round and hard like a gritty potato. "It's a head," I announce with relief, sure of myself now. "And I swear it has hair!"

"Boy or girl?" Frog asks, deadpan. *He's got to be kidding.*

I probe around some more, trying to estimate the width of the cervix, the elastic opening of the uterus. Jody is patient with me but when I feel the head push down during a contraction she moans. The cervix thins and I feel it now. My fingers can open about the width of a small tangerine, about six centimeters, more than halfway. I pull out and wash at the sink. "Frog, sit on the bed and hold Jody's hand or do something useful."

"I'll get some wood."

"No, you hold her hand. *I'll* get the wood!"

HAWK

I throw on my coat, needing fresh air to think. If we don't get moving, this baby's going to come. Outside, there's a clear lavender sky and a quarter moon rising. It will be dark soon and will take us almost two hours, across slush-covered country roads, to get to Two Harbors.

There are closer hospitals in Duluth, but I know for certain that if we go to St. Luke's or St. Mary's, the birth will turn into a medieval torture scene. Frog and I will be pushed aside and Jody whisked away into the white bowels of the hospital. She will be splayed out, flat on her back, on a delivery table in a sterile operating room, her legs up in stirrups, her arms and hands tied down, surrounded by strangers.

I told the couples in my childbirth class to stay home as long as they could, but we may be cutting it too close. To get my friends out of this shack will take momentous effort. It would be easier to let Jody stay here. As she says, this is the way women have been having babies for millions of years. She's young and healthy . . . *but if something bad happens . . .*

I lean my forehead against a tree for strength and take in a big breath, then I load my arms with split cedar, stomp into the shack, and dump the firewood on the floor with a crash. I have no idea if this will work, but I must try.

"Frog," I say with authority, "go warm up the truck." The man stares at me like I'm the bad witch from Oz. "I mean *now!* Take any money you've got stashed. We're going to Two Harbors Hospital."

⁂

In an hour and a half, the lights of the small lakeside town come into view. "I have to push!" Jody growls and grips my hand.

"It's the first stoplight, Frog. Turn left and pull into the hospital entrance. Don't push yet, Jody! It's not time. It can't be time. You'll tear your cervix. Blow, like this."

Frog runs a red light, turns wide with a screech, and we're under the emergency room canopy.

⁂

"Blow, Jody. Blow." I get in Jody's face while the delivery-room nurses pull off her skirt. "The doctor will be here any minute." Frog is mute, transfixed by the row of gleaming silver instruments arranged on the sterile table. "Blow, Jody."

The delivery room doors swing open and Dr. Leppink, in scrubs,

48 Patricia Harman

with a pale green surgical hat and a cloth mask over his lower face, steps in with confidence. He pulls on his latex gloves and sits down on a rolling stool. "It's OK now," he says softly. "Urge to push?"

With Jody's next effort, the top of a small hairy head peeks out. Three contractions later, a red wrinkled infant lies in the OB's arms.

A nurse wraps the baby in a white flannel blanket and hands it to Jody. I stand in the back of the delivery room with my arm around Frog as he wipes his tears. The light is now golden and a string quartet plays in my mind, music of holiness.

ꙮ

"You've got a nice healthy boy." Leppink grins at Jody. He strips off his gloves and shakes hands with Frog, then jerks his head to one side and indicates I should follow him. He's not smiling now.

We stand in the green-tiled corridor. "Patsy, you convinced the nurse she's my patient, but I've never seen her before."

I flinch, my mouth dry. "I *know*. I tried to get Jody to make an appointment, but your secretary said she'd need money up front and she didn't have it. I told her you'd make some arrangement, but when she called back, the woman said you were booked. Jody got discouraged and never tried again."

I'm talking fast now, trying to make my excuses. "When I ended up at her house today and found she was in active labor, with no one to care for her, I took a chance you'd come if they called you, otherwise she was going to have it at home and I'd be in deep shit. I'm no midwife." I cringe at my language and wait for his reaction, staring up at him. He's a tall, graying Scandinavian with a long face, a ringer for the actor who played Death in the Swedish movie *The Seventh Seal*.

Leppink shakes his head. "Well, she made it. Any later and you *would* have been a midwife. I'll talk to her tomorrow about the charges." He moves away, his shoulders stooped, but turns back, raising his eyebrows. "When you think about it, the delivery didn't take more than ten minutes. I'll give them a break on my fee."

The way things turned out, I thought afterwards, we could have had the baby at home, but you never know . . . There might have been a cord around the neck or some other complication. You never know . . . do you?

They named the baby Hawk.

CHAPTER 8

Sap Rising

Daylight and dark now reign equally after six months of Minnesota winter. Stacy and I both suffer the shits again and are having a hard time getting along. I blame myself for not boiling the water, but we've never had trouble before.

At night in bed, we curl away from each other, read our separate books, *Walden* by Henry David Thoreau for me, *Living the Good Life* by Helen and Scott Nearing for him. Then we blow out the kerosene light. Everything irritates. The scrape of a spoon on a plate, the thud of firewood dropped on the floor. We're polite but distant, play with Mica but don't play together.

The problem is we're *together* all the time, cramped in this little log cabin. We've forgotten what we love about each other and we're restless. This must be what the old-timers call cabin fever.

※

"Want to go out in the woods and help me tap the sugar maple trees?" Stacy suggests after breakfast. For days he's been sitting near the cookstove, whittling spouts from white ash tree limbs. Mica plays in the shavings at his feet.

"OK."

All morning, we wander through the forest, searching for maple trees that are at least eight inches across. Here and there, new shoots of life, the tips of pale skunk cabbage and fiddlehead fern, reach for the sun. Stacy whistles while he works. *'Tis a gift to be simple . . . 'Tis a gift to be free . . .*

As the sun sails over the tops of the trees, we hike back to the cabin. Our shoulders bump and we don't pull away. When Mica finally takes his nap, Stacy sits down on the bed beside me and unbraids my hair. He combs it out with his fingers. I reach for him and feel warmth rush through my body, like sap rising in the maple trees . . .

Company

"They let me out for good behavior," Colin laughs. "Really they just wanted to get rid of me." His blue eyes twinkle and his shoulder-length golden hair is tied back in a ponytail. Brilliant, beautiful, and unattached, our old comrade Colin, from the Committee for Non-Violent Action in Connecticut, has just been released from Chicago's Cook County jail. It's been months since we've seen him. I'd just sent a letter to the prison, and now he's here.

"Come here, Baby Bear. How are you and Mama and Papa Bear doing in this little cabin in the woods?" He reaches affectionately for his favorite baby, now two years old. Mica pulls Colin's soft golden beard.

After breakfast, the three of us work next to the cabin in comfortable silence, setting up a maple sugar evaporating pan that Barney lent us. We carry big rocks from the river to support the metal container and then level the pan one foot above the earth for the fire that will burn underneath it.

Snow languishes in patches under the dark balsam and spruce, but otherwise it's mud everywhere. We squish across the saturated earth. Down the hill, the Lester rises over its banks, carrying white foam and loose branches down to the lake.

"Did you hear that the North Vietnamese began a new offensive?" Colin catches us up on the news at dinner. We haven't been to town, so we listen attentively. "More than twenty thousand troops crossed the border into South Vietnam, forcing the South Vietnamese army into retreat. Nixon responded with heavy bombing and by mining Haiphong Harbor. This weekend there'll be demonstrations all over the country. That's why I want to get down to the Twin Cities. Do you want to come?"

I look hopefully at Stacy.

"Can't," Stacy answers. "Once we start maple sugaring we've got to keep going."

Colin cuts off a huge chunk of cornbread and slathers it with apple butter. It's clear he's disappointed.

At dawn, Colin dresses and pulls on his backpack. He just got here but he's already leaving. We hike with him, through the mist, across the Jacobsen's wet eighty acres, to the Jean Duluth Road, where he'll hitch into Duluth, catch Highway 35, and hopefully be in the Twin Cities by noon.

At the blacktop, the three of us, with little Mica on Stacy's back, stand in a circle with our arms around each other. "Be safe," I whisper, knowing my request will fall on deaf ears. Colin will continue to live without thoughts of his own mortality, like a boulder rolling along the rim of a cliff. I would ask him to stay at the homestead, but I know he won't; he must keep moving, a general of a nonviolent army urging on his troops.

Whenever someone leaves us, I worry that he or she will stick out their thumb, get into a vehicle, and never be seen again. I throw my arms around our good friend, hold on tight, and he doesn't pull away. I know he misses us, as we miss him.

When the first vehicle comes into view, Colin waves his arms above his head like he knows the driver. Stacy and I, to improve his chances, disappear like Chippewa Indians into the mist. Then we hurry home, hand in hand, across Jacobsen's foggy field.

Though patches of snow still litter the ground, pale green willows are poised to unfold. Five bufflehead ducks, with their bold black-and-white feathers, rise from the ponds.

Heron

The Lester River now roars with chunks of ice past our cabin, spilling over its banks, dragging debris and fallen trees to Lake Superior. Since our house is on a rise, there's no danger of flooding, but on the other side, in the lowlands, among the cedar and black ash, the water spreads in lesser tributaries everywhere. The power of the rushing river takes my breath away, makes me feel small.

In Duluth today, there's a local demonstration against war taxes at the IRS building and a women's meeting at the university, but we can't go. Even if we *could* find a safe way to get across the water, we must always be cutting and chopping wood.

I find myself reliving Jody's birth all the time, the smells and the sights and the sound of Hawk's first cry. One moment I'm high from that memory and the teeming life all around me, the lift in the spring air, the new buds on the trees, and the next I'm slouching on our bed, staring down through the window at the snarling river and wondering what the hell I'm doing here. I feel like crying all the time, but can't think of a good enough reason. Our isolation bears down on me all the more since Colin hitched away on the Jean Duluth Road.

Day in and day out it's just Stacy, Mica, and me. I sew on my patchwork quilt. I write in my journal. I make beaded necklaces to sell at the co-op. I work on my outline for my childbirth classes some more and contemplate how I could do a regular series like the ones Stacy and I attended in Minneapolis. I could charge a small fee. The difficulty would be, as always, the weather, our lack of transportation, and my responsibilities at the farm.

On my way to the outhouse, thinking these thoughts, I'm startled by the harsh, metallic cries of three great blue herons rising up from the river. As the huge birds fly over, only ten feet above my head, I can make out the delicate lines on their feathers, see their yellow legs dangling, and feel the rush of air under their six-foot wingspan. An ancient Ojibwa saying captures my feelings: *Sometimes I go about pitying myself, and all the while I'm being carried by a great wind across the sky.*

CHAPTER 9

Drowning

Spring is on a roll and there's so much to do in the garden, but we're almost out of money, down to our last twenty-two dollars and fifty cents. This time, when we go into Duluth, we feel like guests at Chester Creek House. In the kitchen I can't find the tea. There's a new Van Gogh print of sunflowers over the mantel. Someone has been storing boxes on our bed.

Stacy strikes out looking for work at the docks and, discouraged, takes Mica back to the homestead early, but I stay to help Jim put together this month's issue of *The Wild Currents*. In the big, nearly empty storefront where we produce our alternative rag, the bare oak boards creak under our feet and the windows are dirty, but the room is warm and soon we bend low over the recycled library tables.

I am at home here and realize how much I miss our political life. For years we were in the thick of things, living at the Draft Information Center, picketing the IRS, handing out antiwar leaflets downtown, helping start the food co-op and the women's support group. As we pursue our dream of subsistence living, our ability to be involved in the revolution fades. It's not that we don't want to, or that our goals have changed, it's just so hard to do both.

Jim types a story about Nixon's law-and-order policies and I finish my article on feminism and the natural-childbirth revolution. I paste down the banner for the newspaper headlines: "Half of All U.S. Citizens Now Oppose War in Vietnam." A political cartoon that Johan Sorensen, my old lover, has drawn goes under the article. I touch the caricature of the president with the tips of my fingers. The action has nothing to do with Nixon; it's Johan I'm reaching for.

※

Three hours later, I stand on the side of the road, hitchhiking alone. I know it's dangerous, but a woman can't let that get in her way. Car after car passes as I watch dark clouds come in from the west, and I'm getting discouraged when finally Mr. Tollefson stops. I toss my canvas knapsack into the bed of his battered blue pickup and jump in.

"Aren't you afraid to hitchhike alone? There's some weird people out here," Tollefson says, shifting his gaze from the road to me. The fleshy growth under his eye quivers. I try not to look at the mole of Lake Superior and answer coolly, "No."

It's a lie. Of course I'm scared, but we have to learn to trust people if we want to make a better world, and besides, I have no other way to get home.

Halfway along, Mr. Tollefson stretches his right arm along the back of the seat, flexing his shoulder, and I respond by sliding closer to the passenger door. Snow flies now, great gobs of it, just as I feared. Thirty minutes of the slap, slap of the window wipers peeling back slush and I point to where I want to be dropped. The wet white already covers the ground. "There by the oak tree."

Tollefson pulls onto the narrow gravel berm. "Your old man at home?"

"He's probably coming across the field to meet me right now," I fib, hoping the old guy will think Stacy's nearby.

"Just wondered," Mr. Tollefson mumbles. "It's getting dark. You shouldn't be out here alone. Don't forget your purse."

I'm hurrying now, more afraid of Mr. Tollefson than I am of the night. As I tromp across the pasture through two inches of slush, the wind scours my face and the wet soaks my hair. I pull my bare hands up into my coat sleeves.

To get to the cabin, I have to hike for two miles across the wind-swept fields and then cross the roaring Lester. When I come to the bank, it's already dusk and I see something bobbing along in the river, churning through the current along with whole small trees. I'm astonished to make out, in the fading light, a deer with a full rack of antlers. The stag struggles to keep its head above water. It flounders and spins.

I run along by its side, helpless to do anything. Where the river curves away through the trees, across the floodplain, the deer is swept under a logjam. The animal turns to me, eyes white with terror, and then he is gone.

❦

I stand staring at the tangled pile of small and large trees where the deer disappeared and then move homeward. At our crossing place, I find the old elm bridge torn away, so, with no other choice, I wade through the shallows in icy water up to my knees. The current is swift and the bottom rocky. Twice I almost fall. Then I crawl up the bank and trod toward the clearing.

"Stacy!" I call. "Stacy." I'm so exhausted and cold, when he finally runs out of the cabin, I burst into sobs. He gathers me in and, when we're inside the cabin, unties my boots. It's only later, as we're getting into bed, that he asks, "What's wrong with you, Patsy? Don't you want to live here? You don't *have* to, you know. No one's forcing you."

Pulling my pink flannel nightgown over my head, I yearn to tell him how hard it was to get home, hitching alone, riding with creepy Mr. Tollefson, hiking across the windy pasture and wading through the icy Lester, but I pinch my mouth shut.

I should be stronger. Shouldn't be such a baby.

As Stacy blows out the kerosene lamp and pulls up the covers, I remember, for the first time, the canvas satchel full of groceries I'd tossed in the back of Mr. Tollefson's pickup. I'd been so anxious to get away from him; I'd forgotten the bag until now. *All our precious provisions from the food co-op, gone!*

Tears wet my pillow. Our quart money jar is empty and we have no funds to replace the lost food. I should reach for Stacy, should ask him to hold me, but that's my trouble; I'm never strong enough . . . . and I'm always trying to be stronger than I am.

I remember the buck being swept down the Lester, unable to get its footing, drowning in water only four feet deep. Its wide eyes roll back as it's pulled under the logjam.

Gift

For three days we hike to the mailbox, hoping the shipment of honey-bees Stacy ordered from the Dadant beekeeping catalog last February will be here. The maples are budding now, small red flowers at the tips of each twig. Trillium, shy, white forest trumpets, are heralding spring, and there's a change in the air, a lift in the light.

Each afternoon, we return from the mailbox empty-handed. We do get a check from the Lakewood Township for $32.45 for overpayment of our land taxes, money we badly need and that cheers us considerably after the loss of our provisions, but still no bees.

Today it's my turn to walk out to the turnaround at the end of Dahl Road, and I don't expect to come home with anything, but Barney calls me over to his front porch. "Little critters finally came. The mailman gave 'em to me. I put them in Ila's work shed." He's dressed in worn, clean coveralls, with a white dress shirt torn at the sleeve.

"Here they are." Barney indicates four containers sitting on the floor by a loom in the neat lean-to attached to the cottage. The boxes have screened sides, and in each buzzing package, a knot of winged insects clusters around another smaller screened box that contains a queen. I stand peering down at them.

"Know what you're gonna do with them?" he asks. "My grandpap kept bees, but he captured the wild ones."

"Stacy learned beekeeping from reading books. He's set up some used hives he bought last summer at the top of the clearing near our little orchard."

Barney reaches for a white cloth flour sack that hangs over the side of the deep concrete sink, and with his big rough farmer hands holds it open. I pick up the four one-pound boxes and place them gingerly in the bag. The hum of the bees goes up a notch. Though they're safe in their screened containers, I handle them with care.

"Oh, and don't forget this." Barney turns. On a hook on the back of the door is my lost canvas satchel. He hands it down. "Lawrence Tollefson left it here yesterday. It's yours isn't it?" I smile, take the bag, and peek in. Everything's there, the pinto beans and cornmeal, the buckwheat flour and precious jar of peanut butter!

🌾

"They came! They finally made it." I hold out the cloth bag of bees as I enter the cabin and lay my satchel on the kitchen counter. Stacy doesn't notice the return of our food supplies, he's so excited about his bees. He jumps up from where he sits on the floor, sharpening the six-foot two-man crosscut saw.

"Are they OK? Do they seem all right?" My lover fusses over them, excited as a boy on Christmas. He extracts each screened box and holds it up to the light.

"They look healthy to me," I answer. "Pretty vigorous . . . though I don't know much about bees."

My companion doesn't know much either. This will only be his second year as a beekeeper. Last summer, on his first attempt, all his bees mysteriously flew off.

As soon as Stacy has safely established the insects, setting the screened cages into the white wooden boxes and opening the tiny doors so the workers can come out, we go up to the garden to turn over new soil. Though we'd had the brief snow flurry a week ago, the temperature's now above seventy.

The alder and willow down by the river have opened their yellow blossoms in the warm morning air. Stacy steps out of his cutoffs and pulls off his T-shirt.

When he strips down, I see that over winter he's lost weight. Sweat beads on his trim, muscular frame. With head down, he slices through the sod while I lean on my hoe and admire his body. Chop. Chop. Chop. He never looks up, just keeps on, like a tireless machine. This is work that he loves and I love it, too, but more moderately.

Inspired, I pull off my jeans and sweater and then take off Mica's clothes as well. Our little boy runs around naked, a natural nudist, with his hands raised wide, yelling, "Yay! Yippee!" as frisky as a newborn lamb. It looks like so much fun, I join him, skipping and leaping into the air. Winter is over; dark is forgotten.

Summer

CHAPTER 10

Wreckage

Dark night. A sliver of moon in and out of the clouds, and I'm nervously singing with gusto all the way home through the woods.

Michael row the boat ashore, hallelujah! Michael row the boat ashore.

The white blackberry blossoms glow in the low light where I cross through the swamp. Stacy is in St. Paul at a War Resisters meeting, so it's just Mica and me. We caught a ride home with Rob after I repeated my childbirth class.

This time there were five couples and two single women. Word is getting around and I tried something new. I asked each person to write down on a slip of paper what he or she was most afraid of. This was a radical innovation. Most childbirth teachers ignore discussing pain, fear, or anything negative, figuring women hear enough of that from their mothers and sisters-in-law. I think differently. It's important to shine a bright light on what haunts us. Shadows are always scarier in the dark.

The fears the participants wrote down were mostly predictable. "I'm afraid of tearing." "I'm afraid I'll let my wife down and won't be a good coach." "I'm afraid of the sight of blood." "I'm afraid I can't take the pain." "What if there's a cord around the neck?" "What if the doctors and nurses get mad at me?" I was able to address the concerns, in a matter-of-fact way, one at a time.

The most difficult fear was, "I worry that I won't be a good parent." There was no way to tell if the handwriting on the little slip of folded paper was a woman's or a man's. I guess we're all afraid of that. You read books by Dr. Spock or A. S. Neill and you think you have a clue, but do we? Do we really?

❄

Michael row the boat ashore, hal . . . le . . . lu . . . jah!

Ever since seeing the big animal tracks down by the river, I've been uneasy in the woods at night. The song gives me courage and warns all porcupine, skunk, bobcat, and *bear* that I'm passing through the woods and they'd better be wary.

At the crest of the hill a scene of destruction assaults me. The white wooden bee boxes in our apiary have all been overturned, the frames of honeycomb scattered; confused bees swarm everywhere. I nearly sink to my knees.

It doesn't take long to figure it out. The bear, or bears, attracted by the scent of honey, have located a pleasure ground.

Friday, before we left for town, Stacy and I had two chores to do *only:* write our articles for *The Wild Currents* and safeguard the hives by building log platforms to protect them from predators. The first chore got done. We both wrapped up our stories.

I wrote about the women's role in the peace movement and used my new pen name, Trillium Stone. Stacy finished his piece on the Vietnam Veterans Against the War. We did our part for the movement but the beehives are gone.

I feel like crying. Instead I swear. "Shit! Shit! *Shit!* Why didn't we build the platform before we left? We are such bunglers!"

"Shit!" echoes Mica.

Stacy loves to lie on his stomach in the tall grass, watching the bees bring in the fuzzy yellow pollen, and they were doing so well. Now the hives are ruined and the colonies destroyed. Mica swivels in his carrier, peering around at the devastation. "Shit!" he giggles again, knowing now that *shit* is a naughty word.

"Look at this, Mica. Stacy's poor bee houses are all gone. It was the bear, I'm sure of it. No *person* would do this. For one thing, they'd be afraid of being stung."

Aimlessly, I wander through the wreckage, picking up the broken honeycomb frames and dropping them again. Insects are buzzing over the bottom of the containers, too stunned to sting. Whether the queens are still alive it's impossible to tell. When I step over the ruined hives,

I feel the sticky stuff under my feet. When I wipe my eyes, I get honey on my face.

In the shadows, a branch snaps and I whip around, but it's only a small animal rustling in the leaves. I'd better get back to the cabin before something big and hairy comes charging out of the woods. It would be hard to run fast with Mica on my back. The rest of the way home, I forgo singing. There's no song for the frustration I feel. In an hour, the fire is crackling and the cabin is comfortable. Mica's fed and asleep upstairs in his homemade bed. I feel bad for the bees but worse for Stacy. He will be so sad when he gets home.

"Well let's do it," I say outloud to the royal *we*. Back down in the kitchen, I unhook the Coleman from the beam and dress myself like a beekeeper, the way I've seen Stacy dress. I even get down his bee hat and veil, and then I march back to the orchard with a jar of maple syrup, on a mission, clanging a soup spoon on the side of the metal lantern to warn the bear I'm coming. Or *bears,* I remind myself. For some reason, I keep thinking there's only one, but I don't know that.

⚘

On the hill, nothing has changed. In the dim light, masses of bees, a disoriented mob, still mill around. Pieces of white wood shine in the lantern's glow and my long shadow almost looks like a bear looming over the scene.

Stumbling through the debris, I discover four intact frames of honeycomb and arrange them in the two damaged boxes that I whack into shape. Finally, I sprinkle some maple syrup around. "Sorry, bees," I say, offering the sweet liquid as an inducement to stay put.

I shake my head slowly and then, leaning back, my arms outstretched, shout into the night, "This means *war,* bears!"

It's a ridiculous threat. We've no guns or traps or even poison. Am I going to meditate them away?

"I mean it!" I shout, as if that settles the matter and they'd better be afraid. I picture them lying in a nearby den, smugly licking their paws and laughing their heads off.

CHAPTER 11

Serfdom

Wild strawberries bloom at the edge of the forest. Fiddlehead ferns reach for the sun. Summer solstice came and went and I threw a few wildflowers into the river to celebrate. Everything's so beautiful on the outside and so not right inside. First there was the bee fiasco. Now the Air Force base up the coast of Lake Superior is practicing bombing raids over the farm.

Day and night, the roar of their engines rips low through our wilderness paradise. First I hear the snarl from across the river and then the jet tears through our airspace, shocks the flowers, shocks the trees, shocks the little cabin in the woods and makes Mica cry.

Nixon has permanently suspended the Paris peace talks, so I guess the pilots need practice before they go back to Southeast Asia and bomb the crap out of everyone. Two days ago, I counted a dozen runs in twenty-four hours.

When we go into Duluth, a photo is plastered all over the papers and on TV. It shows a little Vietnamese girl, completely naked, her clothes torn off because of a napalm attack, crying in terror, with U.S. soldiers, carrying rifles, casually walking behind her.

Once I was a believer in the red, white, and blue. With the war in Vietnam, the assassination of the Kennedy brothers, and the shooting of Reverend King, Old Glory has faded. It hasn't just faded; it's been torn down. To top off everything, when I went up to the garden this morning, I discovered that rabbits had eaten our new cabbage.

"Do you think we should get a guard dog?" I ask Stacy while we eat lunch out in the meadow at our homemade picnic table. "He could watch over our crops, the cabin, and the beehives when we're in town." My lover looks at me as he slurps up the rest of his soup, then wipes his mustache with his hands.

"What would you do, tie him up? Leave him here by himself for days when we went into Duluth? Who would feed him? *What* would we feed him? We can't afford dog food."

"Maybe he could hunt," I offer lamely. I obviously hadn't considered the details.

"Doggie," yells Mica, bashing his spoon on the table. "Doggie!" At least someone is on my side.

❧

Recently we've even discussed purchasing a used vehicle so we could make shorter, more frequent trips to town, but we have no savings. To get that kind of cash, we'd have to move into Duluth, rent an apartment, and pay utilities. That would mean paying taxes for war as well as leaving the homestead vulnerable.

Our goal is to live lightly and sustainably on the earth, to take only what we need, to revere nature, to divorce ourselves from the military-industrialist empire; but I'm weary of living like medieval serfs. Worse than serfs. We don't even have an animal to pull a cart. *Come to think of it, we don't have a cart.*

Thief

A string of days, like lapis and jade on a golden cord. The dark blue Minnesota sky, the deep emerald fields of midsummer, the yellow goldenrod.

Dawn, and the sky is just turning white and I roll over in bed, spoon around my lover, ready to return to sleep, but the sound of distinct scratching on the front door arouses me. The first thing I think is, *it's some passing dog,* although we've never seen a stray out this way before. I picture one of Rob's canines and shuffle, barefoot in my birthday suit, to the window to look down. A black bear squats on our porch, gazing around in the pale morning light.

"Stacy!" I hiss. "We've got company!"

My lover hoists his head.

"Come over. Look!" Pointing down, I'm as excited as a kid at a zoo. The bear turns his black head as Stacy leans over me.

"Where?" my companion asks, rubbing the sleep out of his eyes. I point straight down on the steps, where a mound of black fur now stands up on its hind legs, sniffing. "Shit! He must smell our food. He's probably the thief that destroyed the beehives." Stacy reaches into the toy box, grabs two of Mica's big wooden blocks and starts clacking them. "Get out of here!" he bellows as he clumps down the stairs.

I follow him, nude, and we both stop and peer through the small window at the shaggy animal, his drooling mouth so close I can smell his foul breath through the crack in the door.

"We've got to get rid of him," Stacy worries. "If he starts thinking this is his feeding station, we're in trouble." The creature drops to four feet again and wags his head, none too swift to depart.

"Shoo!" I holler as I grab a metal soup spoon and pull a pot off its nail, banging them together. "*Shoo!*" The beast backs off the porch, glares at the window, then licks his chops. That ticks me off and I throw the door open, almost hitting him. "I *mean* it! Shoo! Get away from our cabin, you fucker! I've about had it with you! I told you this was war!"

I'm standing, *naked,* six feet from a huge black bear, banging on a saucepan. "Shooooooh!" I holler again. The bear ambles leisurely down the trail toward the spring and then stops and looks back, his or her round ears silhouetted in the golden morning dawn, each hair on fire.

Suddenly the animal appears friendly to me, gentle and curious, and I'm half-ashamed I called him fucker—I was only trying to shout something nasty . . . as if he'd be insulted, his feelings hurt. Then I remember the bees and the destruction of the hives and get mad again.

Pounding on my soup pot, I chase the bear down the path. "Get away from here. This is *our* den! Shoo . . . I mean it! I'm serious!" Stacy is standing on the porch, laughing his head off at this hippie version of *I Love Lucy,* sans clothes. He's doubled over, he's laughing so hard. Mica, in his blue footy pajamas, watches with big eyes as his wild, butt-naked mother chases a four-hundred-pound bear through the woods.

CHAPTER 12

Celebration

In the dim evening light, two Canada geese fly low overhead and land in our swimming hole, honking. "Hello, geese!" I call out. "On your way south? Where's the rest of your gaggle?" Just the sound of the word *gaggle* amuses me.

"Hello, geese," Mica echoes from his baby carrier on Stacy's back.

We're heading upriver, on our way to Duluth for the Full Moon Party at Chester Creek House. This August celebration is an important community event, a mark in the North Country calendar that says we made it through another year. The black trunks of maple and poplar are outlined against the fading lavender sky.

"Oh, I forgot to tell you," Stacy says over his shoulder as we crunch through the woods. "When we saw Colin at the conference in Madison, he said he's coming to Minnesota again. He's bringing some friends, people he's met in his travels. They're interested in community."

"A commune here?" I'm afraid to get my hopes up. Stacy and I have lived in four intentional communities in six years, the last one Chester Creek House. Like many hippies, we're searching for utopia, me more than him. When Stacy puts his roots down, he's hard to pull up.

"I don't know about *here*. He just wants us to meet them." We stand on the muddy bank, looking down at the Lester. After days of pounding rain, the river again spills over our log bridge. The far end is already submerged by twelve inches of water.

"What do you think?" Stacy questions. "If we go upstream, we can still get across at the shallow place."

"Let's do it!"

We skip and hop across Jacobsen's field, dancing with our moon shadows, singing the Cat Stevens song, and the stars in Orion's belt are lined up right because within twenty minutes a blue sedan pulls off in the gravel.

At Chester Creek House, the Full Moon Party is in high form. In the side yard, a huge bonfire leaps over the music. Shadows dance on the clapboard house walls and the air smells of cider and wood smoke.

Jody Innis, with baby Hawk, is there, but I don't see Frog. Two women from my last childbirth class come over to greet me. One is the single woman who didn't have a coach. Jody is going to help her. I rub my pregnant friends' bellies and give them a hug for good luck, wishing I could do more, be there to guard them from harm, be there to encourage them.

There's Patrick, bouncing a Bender child on each knee, wearing a red, white, and blue McGovern sweatshirt. Leila is dancing with Courtney, their hands raised over their heads like reeds and their long skirts swirling. Jerry and Joan Bender are passing a beer back and forth.

The full moon shines down on Lake Superior while Jimmy flails away on his guitar and everyone's singing *Bye, bye Miss American Pie* . . . I look around at these good friends and wonder, if we wanted to come back, would there be room for us?

Visitors

Squash gone, tomatoes gone. "Goddammit!" Stacy leans on his hands and knees, breathing heavily. "Why didn't we at least pick the green tomatoes before we went to Duluth? We could have put them in boxes in the window to ripen." We stare around at the mushy orbs drooping from the blackened vines. "Or if we'd just brought in the summer squash . . . Shit! We should have known. We're such screwups."

Because of the Indian summer, for three days we lingered in town after we put out *The Wild Currents*. Aaron was able to get Stacy work at the docks, since he now has an in with one of the foremen, a Vietnam vet who Aaron interviewed for the paper. While Stacy worked unloading heavy crates, I boxed up our linen, town clothes, and books in our old basement room.

One of Jenny and Patrick's friends, Sister Katherine, another teacher, is joining the community and they need the space. I started to roll up our worn oriental rug and then thought better of it. The cement floor looked so cold and bare.

Before we headed back to the farm, Patrick told us we could still crash upstairs in the living room whenever we need to . . . but it won't be the same. The three of us, Mica, Stacy, and I, are on our own now, adrift, without community, without shelter from the storm.

My lover kicks a tomato stake, and the whole bush, withered red and green tomatoes and all, topples over. "We lost our first planting with the late frost in June and now our fall harvest is ruined by an early frost in August. Shit! We gotta get our priorities straight."

"Shit," yells Mica, and I flinch.

"It wasn't the *whole* harvest."

"Halloooo," comes a voice from the other side of the clearing. Colin and four scruffy hippies come through the trees. Colin's golden hair and beard shine in the sunlight and he flashes a wide smile. "Did you say *'shit'*?" he reaches for Mica, his favorite nephew. "I didn't know you could swear!" Mica laughs at the joke, though he doesn't know the word *swear*.

"Hey," Stacy says, giving our friend a stiff hug, embarrassed that the others have heard him freaking out. I'm not so reserved. I throw my arms around Colin's neck, squeezing hard. It is *so* good to see him. He's dressed in the same pale blue denim work shirt that he always wears, tucked neatly into clean jeans, with white canvas sneakers.

We lead the newcomers down through the balsam grove and they gaze with amazement at our hand-built house. I admire the scene from their eyes, this tall sturdy log cabin in the middle of these sparkling woods. It's a picture from a storybook, the flashing river tumbling below, the blue sky above, the wind showering the air with twirling gold leaves.

Colin introduces the guests. "How you doing." "Nice place." "Thanks for having us . . ."

There's a short, bouncy all-American type with apple cheeks, Mara, from Iowa, green bandana knotted around her neck. And Kaitlin from

Detroit, dark tan, white teeth, wearing an embroidered peasant shirt and jeans.

There's Tristan, an intense Norseman from Indiana, over six feet four, with a shock of red hair and a beard to match, and another thin, quiet guy in a worn tie-dyed T-shirt. Tom, I think that's his name.

❧

"Stacy and Patsy are the most self-sufficient homesteaders I've met," Colin tells the group after dinner as we lounge around the campfire up in the big clearing, our feet stretched out to the flames.

"What we're doing here is experimenting with voluntary poverty," Stacy explains. "We choose to live as two-thirds of the world's poor live. We're trying to answer the question: can we find a way to live sustainably? Not just us, but the generations that will come after us." He lays his hand for a moment on Mica's blond head to make his point.

"Industrialized countries are polluting the environment and using up the resources that belong to our children and their children. See, it's all connected."

"How does *community* fit in?" Tom asks.

Stacy takes a big breath, looks at me, and goes back to his carving.

"We've lived at four or five communes . . ." I take up the story he doesn't want to tell. "But finding the right community is even harder than living sustainably. So far, at each place, we've made good friends, but the balance wasn't right. We met Colin at the Committee for Non-Violent Action, but that was too scary to me."

"Like what?" Mara asks.

"Like violence and the threat of violence. One night a bunch of drunks came down the gravel drive in pickups, hung around outside for hours in the dark, yelling 'Go home commies!' We crouched in the dark kitchen, not knowing what they would do. I thought we would die. In the end they fired shotguns into the windows and left.

"Another time, one of our guys was beat nearly senseless at a vigil at the nuclear-powered submarine base at Norwich. Ended up in intensive care. Almost didn't make it. The cops don't care. They figure if we protest, we're on our own. A month later, the thugs tried to burn down our outbuildings. Very hostile territory. Too hostile for me."

"You're the rural arm of the revolution," comforts Colin.

Maybe. If you can call an isolated farm in the middle of the Minnesota backwoods a revolution.

❦

"It's getting late. I'd better put Mica to bed." I lean over Mara, holding out my hands for my little boy. "Come on, baby." I'm surprised when Mara silently follows me down to the cabin. She pushes the heavy door open for me.

"You don't have any sanitary pads do you?" she asks. I pull Mica's red mittens off and throw them on the window seat. She's putting the kettle on the cookstove. The question embarrasses me.

"Geez, no. I just use menstrual rags and wash them out. Saves on paper and trees." I'm sure the woman will think I'm gross, but she responds without blinking. "Great. I'll wash them down at the river and give them back clean."

I find my stack of torn white cloths, folded in a shoebox under the sink, and hand them over. Mara sits down on the window seat, watching me wrestle Mica into his pajamas.

"You like having a baby?"

"I do. I don't know what I expected. I was never one of those girls that couldn't wait to be a mom, but it's comfortable."

"I'd like to have kids, but I'd be afraid to give birth. The whole idea . . . a baby coming out of my vagina! Maybe I'll adopt. Did it hurt? They say it's terrible."

I shake my head. "I haven't had much pain in my life, but it's not like getting your arm cut off. It's a different kind of pain, and if you know what to expect, it's not bad. . . . I mean, my labor was long and hard and it hurt more than I imagined, but I survived. You could do it . . . . You just have to get your mind out of the way; your body knows what to do."

"Get your mind out of the way?"

"Yeah, don't think too hard. Stacy and I spent months of preparation, like we were working out for a marathon. I must have read ten books, everything from *Thank You Doctor Lamaze* to *Childbirth without Fear,* and we went down to the Twin Cities for childbirth classes eight times.

"I looked everywhere for a midwife, but the only one in the state is eighty years old, charges four hundred dollars, and won't leave Minneapolis. I visited the director of nursing at both of the hospitals in Duluth but neither allow the father to be present or let you deliver naturally, so we drove thirty miles to a little hospital up the coast.

"In the end, we didn't get a perfect birth but a good one. Stacy was my rock, and I know, for us, all that preparation was worth it, but if we'd just had a midwife, someone to be our guide, I bet we could have done better. Like I said . . . you just have to get your mind out of the way . . . the body knows what to do."

Mara leans over and gives Mica a hug. "Maybe . . . Maybe I could do it. I guess I could. He looks worth it."

Later, lying on my back under the quilts after I've tucked Mica in, I smile, hearing voices rise from the clearing and remembering the relaxed, hopeful faces. *There is a season, turn, turn, turn . . .* I can just make out Mara's soprano, Kaitlin's alto, Tristan's bass, and Colin's tenor. Stacy and Tom are both baritones. *A time for every purpose under heaven.*

Baptism

At breakfast, the kitchen smells of oatmeal, cinnamon, and maple sugar. There's a body on every surface in our little log house, the window seat, the four chairs, even the floor. Sunlight streams through the west window. *Morning has broken, like the first morning,* Mara sings as she wipes off the kitchen counter. *Blackbird has spoken, like the first bird . . .*

I study these people carefully, wondering what it would be like to live with them. There's no doubt we all care about building a new world, but what kind of builders would they be? Would they tirelessly cut and drag wood from the forest? Dig holes for fruit trees? Climb up in the wind to fix the roof? And what are they like when they're hungry? And what are they like when they're tired and hot?

For lunch, after working on the root cellar, we arrange a picnic on blankets down by the swimming hole. The day has turned warm and it's fall equinox, though it still feels like summer. Cumulus clouds float overhead and the leftover maple leaves glitter in the midday light. Winter will be upon us soon, but Stacy strips off his clothes and dives, with a shout, into the chilly water.

The rest of us follow, pulling off jeans and T-shirts. Our bodies are thin and muscular, some tanned, some pale as a ghost, but no one's too shy to go skinny-dipping. I realize, once more, how lonely I am for community.

Mara and Kaitlin break out into song, an old spiritual. *As I went down to the river to pray, studying about that good old way, and who shall wear the robe and crown* . . . We all pick up the gospel song and pretend to baptize each other, playing like kids. I push Tom's head under the water. Then he dunks me.

I let myself float on my back with my arms wide open and the current carries me downstream, away from the voices. The Lester is clean and metallic. Above me the branches bow over my head. It's a river of light, I think, a river of rainbows.

Summer Camp

By the end of the week, a stack of split logs as high as my chest is piled against the side of the cabin. The root cellar now has shelves, a roof, and a door. Our friends are leaving in the morning and our last bonfire is like the closing session of summer camp. We sit in the grass or on logs, in a tighter circle now. Mica is wrapped inside Kaitlin's jacket so only his blond head peeks out under hers, his white fuzz surrounded by her long dark hair. Tristan lies on his sleeping bag with his head on Mara's lap. Tom has taken up whittling.

Colin speaks for us all, like the camp chaplain. "This has been a good week, a time for reflection and labor, a time to get to know each other. I hope we can continue this fellowship and work together in the future." He's referring not just to the chopping of wood, the singing of songs, and the frolicking in the river, but the meetings we had, each day, to discuss our dreams of community and how we might actualize them.

"Amen," Kaitlin whispers. I peek over at Stacy to see what he's thinking. He rests next to Mara, smiling into the flames. Golden sparks shower up like fireworks when Tom carefully drops another log on the flames.

Later, in bed, I pull up the quilt against the chilly evening, curl around my lover, and whisper into the dark. A shaft of silver moonlight comes from the window. "They're nice aren't they?"

"Mmmmm."

I can't tell if that's a yes or a no. "I really like them. Don't you?" I want Stacy to answer, *Yes, these are our people.* But he rolls on his back and stares up at the beams.

"Tom and Tristan seem to be hard workers. Colin has the vision." That's all he says, then his breathing slows and I know he's asleep.

❦

In the morning, frost covers everything. Cobwebs are beaded with tiny balls of ice and the berry bushes sparkle. Every leaf and blade is rimmed with white. As Stacy, Mica, and I help our friends roll up their tents and then escort them to their truck at the end of Dahl Road, we walk on crystal.

"Well, good-bye, man." Stacy offers Colin one of those guy hugs. They pat each other's backs.

With wet eyes, Colin ruffles Mica's corn silk hair. "'Bye, little buddy." When my turn comes, I hold Colin fiercely. His beard smells of soap and the campfire. I have loved him for years, loved his body, loved his mind, loved his courage, maybe not the way he loves me, but no matter. He returns my squeeze and gives me a buzz on the neck that gives me goose bumps.

Tom helps Mara climb into the bed of the pickup, where they settle against their packs. Kaitlin, Colin, and Tristan scramble into the cab. "See you at the Peacemakers conference in Cincinnati," Colin reminds us, leaning out the passenger window.

"We'll see . . ." Stacy responds. "I doubt we can both come. I hate to leave the homestead for long. Last winter we had those vandals . . ."

Kaitlin blows us a kiss. Mara waves and Tom reaches out as the truck pulls away. Our fingertips touch.

Then Stacy and I, hand in hand, with Mica swinging between us, walk slowly down through the swamp, where dried ferns catch in our bootlaces, up through the tiny, now naked, orchard, past the beehives, and finally into the clearing, bigger than when we left, emptier.

Fall Again

CHAPTER 13

Dilemma

"Sorry I got here so late," Wren apologizes when she meets me at Leif
Erickson Park. When I saw her at the food co-op she asked me to meet
her here alone on this warm autumn day, so I knew something was up.
The tall twenty-eight-year-old pulls her one long braid back and refas-
tens the rubber band. She's a thin woman with shiny dark hair, a wide
smile, and straight teeth. "I just needed to talk to you alone. I found out
last week that I'm pregnant."

"Yeah?" I bend down and take Mica out of his baby carrier so he can
run around. Wren is a senior at the University of Minnesota, Duluth.
We haven't seen that much of each other since she went back to school
to major in early-childhood education. I can tell by her voice that this
is bad news.

"I think I should get an abortion," she continues. The word sounds
like metal dropping down a laundry chute. I watch Mica chase a flock
of pigeons across the lawn, his fine blond hair blowing.

"You think?" Politically I'm pro-choice, but I've never really known
anyone who's had a termination, don't even know where they go. How
do I reconcile abortion with my pacifism? Fortunately Wren doesn't ask
me what she should do or what I would do if I wore her shoes. "Who's
the dad?"

"That's part of the problem. I don't know. I broke up with John. I
told you about that. He was fooling around with that waitress at the
country club where he works as a cook. Then I got together with Louis,
a guy in my psych class. I really liked him, but John started calling,
wanted to make a new start, and you know, we'd lived together for
four years, so I thought I should try. Somewhere during that time I must
have forgotten one of my birth control pills . . ." There are tears in her

76

brown eyes. I reach over and take her hand as we follow Mica down the gravel trail toward the gazebo.

"I don't know what else to do. John and I weren't back together more than two weeks until we started fighting and he moved out again. He's not daddy material, that's for sure, and I hardly know Louis. I don't have any money and my parents told me when I left Kansas that I was burning my bridges. If I have the baby, I won't be able to finish my degree. I've gone over the whole thing three hundred times and don't see any other option. I've weighed everything back and forth and I feel like I'm going crazy."

All around us the last roses of summer bloom in the formal gardens, red, yellow, and peach. I don't find anything surprising about Wren's behavior or how she thinks. I've had more than one lover at a time. I've done my share of dumb things. I just wish she didn't have to face such a decision. Wren would make a good mom . . .

"Have you talked to John and what's his name, Louis?"

"No. Can you imagine how complicated *that* would be? I was only with Louis a few times, and John will freak out, just make things worse. He'll want to take responsibility, but he's such a flake. I'm alone in this."

We lean against the rail of the gazebo, watching the water of Lake Superior lap up on the shore, white foam like lace on the sand. I frown, thinking of Stacy and what a good dad he is. How would he feel if I terminated his baby without even telling him? Mica is arranging stones along the gazebo steps. Once he was only a few cells in my womb. Where does life begin and end?

Despite the beauty around us, the roses, the light, the sound of the waves, this day has turned dark.

There's no scale of justice in our hearts to weigh a decision like this and I have no wisdom to offer, no lifeboat in a storm, nothing but my body, so I take Wren in my arms and rock her, rock her back and forth like a baby, while she looks down at Mica and cries. A seagull cries with her, high in the wind.

Lost

Hard freeze, last night, but it warms up fast. After a lunch of lentil soup and homemade whole-wheat bread, Stacy and I go up to the big clearing to tend our remaining fall crops: kale, cabbage, and a few drooping rutabaga. We sit Mica down at the edge of the garden, in the tall yellow grass, where he can entertain himself with his bag of blocks and sock monkey.

I stare at the ring of dirt and burned branches where our campfire was three weeks ago, a charred reminder of our new friends, a wound in the soil, but more than that, a wound in me, a hole where there wasn't one before. My loneliness seems deeper since Colin and the others bumped away in the pickup. I think of their voices, singing around the flames, and start to cry. I'm so sensitive. Something is wrong with me.

Stacy seems as stalwart as ever. Though the day has a chill, he's thrown off his shirt, and his bare, tanned back gleams with sweat. He churns through the soil, singing with pleasure. *I'm gonna jump down turn around, pick a bail of cotton. Gonna jump down turn around pick a bail of hay* . . . Chop. Chop. Chop. I pick up my hoe and join him. It's hard to be sad on such a beautiful day, with such a joyful companion. *Gonna jump down turn around* . . .

☼

A few minutes later I lean back, wipe my face, and glance around. "Where's Mica?"

My companion shades his eyes. "He was over by you playing in the dirt a minute ago."

I drop my garden tool and move around the near end of the clearing. Stacy goes back to tilling the soil. Chop. Chop. Chop.

"Mica," I call, stooping to peer under the sumac bushes, with their burning red leaves. "He's not here, Stacy."

"Well, he's probably back at the cabin."

I trot back through the balsam grove and circle our house. "Mica!" I call again. At first, like Stacy, I'm not worried. Our little boy has never gone away from us before. How far could a two-year-old go?

Then I think of the river. I race around the two-story building, peer between the trunks of the maples into the nearly naked woods, and run down the hill to the Lester. The ripples glint sinister in the harsh afternoon sun, slash me like a sword. *Shit.* I can't find him! He's vanished. Now I'm sick to my stomach.

"Micaaa!" I shout. I'm not sure what to do, so I run back up the hard dirt path, through the balsam grove to the meadow.

"Stacy!" He's only thirty yards away, but the wind blows in the wrong direction. "*Stacy!*" Finally, he turns. "Mica's *not* at the cabin. Come on. You've got to help find him!"

"What?" Still he can't hear. He drops his hoe and ambles barefooted toward me, the legs of his jeans rolled up to his knees.

"You've got to help me find him."

"What?"

"Mica's *gone,* I tell you. I can't find him anywhere!"

"Where'd you look?"

"All around both clearings, in the chips by the woodpile, and down by the water."

When I mention water, Stacy immediately understands the danger and sprints for the river. The Lester is now five feet deep in front of the house, even deeper down by the swimming hole. If Mica slipped off the bank, he could be a quarter mile downstream by now, lifeless as the deer trapped under the logjam.

"Mica! Micaaa!" we both scream.

"OK, let's not panic," Stacy says when he comes back to the cabin. "He could be anywhere. Let's be systematic. He's never gone near the river by himself before. What's most likely?"

I stare wildly around, trying to think. How could I let this happen? I should have been watching my precious boy! A mother *always* knows where her baby is. *I should have been watching.*

"He can't be in the house, the door is too heavy and the handle too high, but I'll look anyway." When I come out without Mica, Stacy is pacing back and forth on the trail.

"Let's check along the riverbank again," he barks. "Except for the bear, that's the most dangerous." *The Bear. I hadn't even thought of the bear!* "You go downstream as far as the swimming hole, then cut over to the orchard. I'll run out toward the swamp. He wouldn't have time to get farther."

"If he hasn't fallen in the river already."

"Patsy, don't even talk like that! Don't even *think* like that." We both run off, barefoot, just as we were when we worked in the garden. I'm sending a prayer out to the universe, *Oh little blond boy, be safe, be alive!*

"Micaaa!" I cry over and over. I hear Stacy's voice shouting too, getting farther away. As I come up the orchard rise, greenbriars snatch at my jeans. Stones cut my feet. My voice is hoarse from yelling but I can't give up.

Be here! Be here! Be here! I pray with each ragged breath, hoping to find our little boy in the bee yard, covered with honey. I don't care if there are bees crawling all over him, just so he's safe.

At the top of the knoll, the four bee houses squat in the sunlight, but there's no Mica anywhere. From the hill I can see into the birch grove, where the narrow white trunks stand like a Greek chorus, accusing me. *How could you let this happen, a mother always knows where her baby is!*

"Micaaa!" I call, turning in the four directions with my hands cupped to my mouth.

"*Micaaaaaaa!*" No answer.

When I stop, the silence engulfs me. There's only the placid buzz of the bees as they come and go with goldenrod pollen covering their legs, and a pileated woodpecker up in a pine, laughing like Woody Woodpecker.

🐝

Now I move more slowly, and for the first time notice my feet. If I knew what to do next, the pain wouldn't matter. I'd run on until I dropped. Our little boy has bare feet too, I remember, and swipe my eyes with the back of my hand.

By the time I stumble down to the cabin, I'm not even yelling Mica's name anymore. I've moved on to thinking what to do next. We'll have to walk out to Rob's and call someone, the police, I suppose. They'll send out a search team, maybe the National Guard or soldiers from the air base, the men I curse when they roar over the farm in fighter jets.

The authorities will glare at us through their metallic shades, thinking us the worst kind of hippies, child neglecters, too stoned or high to take care of our kid. They'll see the primitive way we live, our clothes, the dirt on our faces. They won't understand that losing my child is like losing my soul, like my heart torn out of me. Then I hear voices.

"Ila gives me cookies," Mica explains, cradled safely between Stacy's knees, his overall jeans rolled up like his father's and his long-sleeved red T-shirt dribbled with food. He kicks his bare feet in the water. "I visit Ila and Barney." Stacy lies on the riverbank, resting back with his head on his hands, gazing up at the last few leaves.

For a moment, I'm furious. How long have they been resting here while I ran frantically through the woods? Then I see Stacy's face, wet with tears.

"We just got home," he offers, pulling me down next to them. "I found Mica in the Olsens' kitchen. He followed the trail all by himself."

"That's over a mile!" I reach over Stacy's legs and give our two-year-old a fierce hug. "You *scared* Stacy and Patsy. Don't ever go away from us again, OK?"

"I told him," Stacy assures, taking my hand.

"Ila gives me cookies," Mica tries to make clear, his blue eyes serious because he knows he's caused us real pain. Our little boy's gaze shifts to and fro, willing us to understand. Then the three of us lie back in the hot sun on the bank of the Lester, listening to the river bubble its way to Lake Superior. Fear has diminished me, and all that's left is the high wind moving the clouds.

Roots

Lately the melancholy flute music is in my head all the time. I'm curled on the window seat, watching Stacy and Mica cook. Stacy is such a wonderful father. He carefully shows his son how to measure brown rice, demonstrates by holding the glass measuring cup up to the light and pointing to the red line. He has Mica add salt and stir the grain in the cast-iron cook pot. Outside the kitchen window, dark clouds have come in.

I gaze at the warm walls of this sturdy log structure, the straight grain of the yellow poplar, the white caulking that keeps out the cold, and wonder what's wrong with me. Stacy and I have been to couples' counseling in Duluth a few times, trying to figure things out, but it's getting us nowhere. The more I talk, the more I appall myself. I don't know what I want and I want everything . . . I have a good man, a secure home, and a beautiful son. What else could there be, communion with saints?

In the afternoon as we harvest potatoes out in the field, this time with Mica secure in his baby carrier, propped in the dirt by our side, I try again to explain my feelings to Stacy. "I know that what we're doing on the land is part of learning to live nonviolently, learning to live sustainably, but while we're out here grubbing around in nature, the war goes on, bloodier than before, people live in poverty, kids are abused . . ."

Stacy turns the soil with his spade but doesn't say anything. He flips over the soil, exposing the brown globes of sweet carbohydrates. I know he's thinking, *She wants to leave again. She wants to go searching for the Garden of Eden.*

I throw my long braids over my shoulder to keep them from dragging in the dirt and crawl behind him, picking out the potatoes with my bare hands and tossing them on a tarp.

"So, what are you saying?" Stacy finally responds.

I take a deep breath. "I don't know . . . maybe we should leave the homestead, just for this winter, hitchhike to California and join the grape boycott or maybe go down to Tennessee, check out Ina May and Steven Gaskins' farm . . . They have midwives there that do home-births. See where life takes us."

Stacy stomps hard on his spade, bites the inside of his cheek, turns the earth over, then steps hard again. "The grape boycott is practically over, Patsy. Anyway, we moved four times in the last few years. I'm tired of it. Every time we settle, you find something wrong and want to move on. It means a lot to me to wake up each morning in the same bed with the sun shining into our cabin at the same angle every day, to see the seasons change in the same way each year. We're just starting to get the garden in shape. I've taken root here."

I let out a long sigh. I know he's right. Wherever we've landed, when we pack up again, it's always my idea. We have a baby together. If he won't leave, then I must stay.

CHAPTER 14

Vision

First snow! Though I dread the hardship and isolation of a long winter,
I can't help it; I'm excited. Stacy loves the snow, too. We run up to the
big clearing and throw our arms wide, raise our bare hands to the huge
white clusters. "Yippee!" I whirl around. Stacy dances a jig and I love
this wild man with all my heart. By afternoon the flurry has turned to
sleet and we realize this is serious weather.

✵

Night comes. We're tired, unprepared for the cold again, and con-
fronted with six months of winter. The unseasonable warmth fooled
us once more. We should have brought in a supply of dry wood and
covered the woodpile with the tarp, but now most of the maple and oak
rounds, stacked against the house, are soggy and wet.

After a quick supper of peanut butter sandwiches on homemade
whole-wheat bread, Stacy builds up the fire in the heater stove and takes
Mica, who's having a meltdown, directly to bed. Outside, wet snow
comes in at an angle and sticks to the stout poplar logs.

Peace I ask of thee, oh river, Stacy sings upstairs, trying to quiet Mica's
tears. *Peace. Peace. Peace . . . When I learn to live serenely, cares will cease.*

That's my problem; I don't know how to live serenely. Nothing's
ever good enough, or what seems perfect at first, sours, like Chester
Creek House, like this homestead. I glance out the window at the frost-
ing covering each branch and twig. Though the hour is early, father and
son fall asleep in our big bed.

✵

The kettle is whistling, so I make myself a cup of hand-gathered peppermint tea and take a chair where I can look out as day turns to dusk,

and white, like a blanket, covers everything. The room darkens, but I don't light the lamp. This will be our second winter on the farm, and our future seems as bleak as the nation's hope for peace. Though at the teach-in I made a convincing attempt to explain simple living as the land-based arm of the revolution, I have my doubts.

There's nothing I love more than floating on my back in the Lester River, my arms stretched out, looking up at the dragonflies glinting metallic-green in the forest light, but what I recall, when I think of my life here, is the intense labor it takes just to survive, from sunup to sundown. Stacy thrives living this way, but I'm not sure this is all I want to do.

Trouble is . . . I don't know what else . . . Teach childbirth classes, maybe, but that's hardly a full-time living, and what about our other goals, trying to live sustainably on the earth, protesting the war, building a new society?

Outside, in the Christmas-card world, snow hangs on every drooping balsam limb, covers rock and tree and stump. I cherish this land, the clearing around the garden, the snake-like path to the spring, the Lester River as it rushes, golden in the sunset, past our home.

I revere every hand-hewed square log in this beautiful cabin, Mica's toy chest painted with blue birds, the window seat with its quilted cover, even the old cast-iron cookstove. It's the way I've always wanted to live . . . or thought I did.

Most of all, I love the dream, the dream of this homestead being a safe haven, a place to raise children with the man I love as we learn to live gently on the earth.

And what about Mica? Mica our cub, sleeping upstairs, with his father's strong arms around him. *What about Mica?* How could I leave?

The room's getting chilly, but movement outside the window draws my eyes to the balsam trees. The wet flakes come down so thick it's hard to see. I lean toward the glass, then freeze, my cup halfway to my mouth. Like a black-and-white photo developing in a chemical tray, the shadow slowly materializes. A large, dark, hairy animal sits under a tree. Our eyes lock. I could wake Stacy to come down and see, but this is personal. It's Fucker, the bear I'd chased down the path last spring. Maybe he's my totem spirit.

"So," I whisper. The bear cocks his head. "What should I do? Go? Stay? Take Mica on the road with me? Join up with Colin, Kaitlin, Mara, and Tom? Leave Stacy alone on the homestead without his boy? How can I do that? I'm a lost soul." The lump of dark fur holds my gaze and tears fall into my peppermint tea. "I don't know what to do . . . *I don't know.*" The bear rubs his back against the trunk, up and down, side to side, as if absently itching a sore spot.

I lay down my mug, expecting the movement to scare the animal away, but it doesn't.

"It will be cold here soon. Shouldn't you be hibernating? Is that what I'm supposed to do, too? Stay here another year, holed up in this log cabin, hiding away?" I think of the isolation, the deep snow, the broken snowshoes, the wet wood, the forty-below nights, the freezing hands.

I can see no way to create community on this isolated homestead. *Who else would want to live this way?* And Stacy won't abandon the land. He's put down roots. These eighty acres of earth make him happy, give him peace. The bear swings his head, snuffs the white that covers the ground. This may be the last time I'll see him.

Upstairs, Stacy stirs in his sleep. I glance at the beamed ceiling, picturing his arms wrapped around Mica. *Peace. Peace. Peace.* The tears start again. When I look back at the balsam grove, the bear's gone.

Gift

Incense and patchouli oil. Rows of green and blue lava lamps. Feathered roach clips and psychedelic posters with peace signs. I'm leaning over the antique counter of the Head Shop on Fourth Street in Duluth, fanning out my macramé necklaces and beaded amulets on the glass surface. A long-haired male clerk, wearing jeans and a white embroidered muslin shirt, bends over the counter, helping me put prices on the necklaces. "If they all sell," he says, "you'll get forty dollars."

Like Silas Marner, I add up the coins in my mind. Forty dollars plus the birthday money that my mom sent will buy a bus ticket south.

"These are beautiful," the clerk goes on in his gentle voice. It's Johan. "They should go fast. We'll hang them on the rack near the register."

He pushes his shoulder-length hair behind his ears and leans his elbows on the countertop. His long, lean body, so different from Stacy's solid, muscular one, stretches next to me.

"You doin' OK?" He places his hand over mine. I go very still. His tenderness overwhelms me and tears start to form, not falling yet, just hanging there.

I shake my head no but answer, "I'm fine." I want him to hold me.

The brass bells on the glass door shatter and cold air comes in. "Hi, babe," bubbles a wispy Tinker Bell. She's Johan's new lover, I'm sure of it, the self-assured way she enters the shop. She doesn't say hello, just flutters to the back, with three cloth bags of food from the co-op, and pushes through the beaded curtain.

"Gotta go," Johan whispers. Then louder, in his shopkeeper's voice, "We'll take the usual ten percent commission, but you'll come out fine. I can mail the check when your necklaces sell or give you cash, next time you come in."

Tinker Bell calls, "Honey? Can you help me put the food away?"

"Thanks," I say, meaning more than just, "Thanks for selling my beaded necklaces."

Thanks for caring. Thanks for loving me once. *The moon and stars were the gift you gave.*

Like a dashing English pilot, I throw my long rainbow scarf around my neck, zip up my parka, and turn toward the door just as three teens in fringed suede jackets push their way in.

"See you." I glance back, wanting to touch Johan's hand once more, but the moment is gone. For a second, he holds my eyes, blue into blue, like rain falling into Lake Superior. Then the door shuts behind me, the brass bells jingle again, and he's gone.

Pilgrim

Sunshine and crisp shadows on old snow. The sound of water dripping everywhere. Winter has temporarily released us, but she will be back again with a heavy boot, to settle her score.

I'm waiting in a wooden shelter for the Sky Line bus that will take us to Jody's new apartment. She and baby Hawk have moved into town. Frog left his shack on Zimmerman for the winter and went down to Minneapolis to work as a roadie for a new Twin Cities rock band.

Tattered political posters flip in the breeze on the back of a nearby phone booth, signs that remind me of the results of the election, and I stand up and rip Nixon's picture down. Not that it will do any good. He won by a landslide and we have four more years of his face to look forward to.

"Come on, Mica. Here's our ride." We stand on the curb and wave to the green city bus that pulls up in the puddle in front of us.

"Hi," Mica greets the driver, holding out his hand for a lift up, and we find seats in the front.

⚘

I finger the crumpled note in my pocket. In his cramped script, our friend Colin has summoned Stacy and me to meet him at the Ohio Peacemakers conference in January. Mara and Kaitlin, Tristan and Tom will be there, along with Tristan's wife, Annie, and some other folks we haven't met from Cincinnati. They're going to discuss forming a new intentional community.

Stacy says he's not going. What would be the point, anyway? He doesn't plan to desert the land. We've come to a standoff. My lover won't consider leaving and I can't envision staying another desolate winter in this Siberian wilderness. That's how I think of the homestead now, as if I've been sentenced to another dark season in the bleak gulag of the North.

My concern is mostly for Mica. Stacy will manage, at least physically, if I leave. He assures me he will, anyway, but would I be breaking his heart? How would I know? His true heart's like the center of a maple tree, full of sweetness, but hard to tap.

"I don't want you to stay unless you *choose* to, Patsy," he tells me. "You aren't a prisoner here. You'll poison this place if you stay without loving it. This way of life brings me joy."

And what about Mica? If I take my boy on the road with me, I won't know from night to night where I'll sleep. I won't know where I'm going until I get there. I won't know what I'll find until I know what I'm looking for. What kind of life is that for a little kid?

Some would say, "Get on with it girl! Quit the whining and self-recrimination." But those people aren't mothers. Those people aren't in love with Stacy. I lie shattered at the bottom of a long mining shaft, covered by rubble. I can't see light, not even a pinpoint.

"Sky Line and Eighth," shouts the driver. This is our stop. Mica and I jump down the steps and trudge through three blocks of slush toward Jody's apartment. The wet snow glitters in the bright afternoon light, but I see none of this. Something massive is shifting, like a glacier sliding over the land.

Dance

A man knocks hard on the bathroom door, rattling the handle. "Come on!" he growls. "The rest of us want showers, too. You're using up all the hot water!" I push my forehead against Jody's slimy shower wall.

In the living room, I can hear Mica telling Jody and Hawk a story about the fox we saw this morning on our way across Jacobsen's field. My little prince . . .

Cat Stevens sings on the stereo, "Morning Has Broken," and the warm iron-tinged water pours down on my face, mixes with my tears. I've been standing in the shower for thirty-five minutes.

"What the fuck!" snarls the deep voice. "Are you coming out, or do I have to come in and get you?" I choke back my sobs.

"Just a few more minutes." The sound of the shower, a little Niagara, muffles my tears. If I walk away, our beautiful wilderness farm and the shining Lester River will be lost to me. For more than two years I have tramped every inch of that piece of earth. It is my earth. I belong there.

"You all right?" Jody questions, sticking her blond head through the door into the steam.

"Just a few more minutes," I repeat my mantra. Something is splitting open inside me, like a baby trying to get born.

Adjusting the shower, I rinse my long hair; turn the temperature to cold and then scalding again. I can hit the road or stay at the farm, but I can't stay in this shower forever. I twist off the spigot.

It is over. After seven years with Stacy, it is over, our love, our travels, our fading dream of building a new world together. There's no telling what will become of us . . . but next week, or maybe the week after, I'll use my small stash, take the Greyhound bus south alone, and meet up with Colin and Mara. I don't know how long I'll be gone or when I'll be back.

Maybe I'll find another farm as beautiful as our homestead, with people who aspire to a better world, men and women who will revere the land and work for peace. In time, maybe I can persuade Stacy to join and he and Mica and I can be together again. This is my hope, a tiny embryo of hope.

I wrap a large white towel around my damp body and step into a narrow hall that smells like marijuana and baking bread. "It's all yours," I say to the scowling bearded guy leaning against the wall.

In the living room, Mica runs up to me, grabs my legs, and unintentionally pulls my towel down. "Tell Jody about the fox, Patsy. Tell her about the fox we saw!"

"Whoops," I laugh as I lift him against me.

I'm naked and damp, standing in a room full of hippies, while President Nixon blabs on a silenced TV, Tricky Dick, telling lies again. No one looks at the commander in chief or at me, either.

You're only dancing on this earth for a short while. Two ponytailed guys and Jody are slumped on the sofa, harmonizing with Cat Stevens and passing a joint back and forth. A sheet of snow roars off the roof. Nude, I swirl Mica around to the music, his arms flung wide. Around and around . . .

We dance until we are dizzy.

✻

Commune on the Ridge

1977–1978

✻

Fall

CHAPTER I

Decision

"Listen, Gracie, and Simon, this isn't false labor. You're leaking fluid and the baby's a month early." I take off my exam gloves and roll them inside out.

I'm sitting on a white chenille spread on a sagging metal bedstead, in the bedroom of a farmhouse sixty miles from our communal farm in West Virginia, one hour, on dirt roads, from the closest hospital. Contractions are moderate and five minutes apart. The patient is six centimeters dilated.

"If we leave for the hospital right this minute, we might make it, or you could be delivering in the pickup by the time we get to the ER in Spencer."

What I'm picturing is, if we make it in time, the scene will be a disaster. The thin thirty-year-old, expecting her first baby, will be assaulted by bright lights and strangers, doctors and nurses, who will flare their nostrils at our strange hippie garb and think Grace a lunatic for trying to have an out-of-hospital delivery. They'll push Simon aside, wheel Grace into the delivery room, strap her down and give her gas as she begs them not to. The couple has been planning a homebirth since before they conceived. Beethoven's *Moonlight Sonata* plays low on the stereo.

"As your midwife, I can go either way, but thirty-six weeks is borderline for delivering at home. The baby will be tiny, maybe five pounds. We'll have to work hard to keep its temperature up and get it to breast-feed . . ."

Grace, a pale, dark-haired woman who trails through life like a silk scarf, teaches piano lessons to children in town. Simon, a thin dropout from MIT with a long, scraggly red beard and a Fu Manchu mustache, works on a hippie carpentry crew. "I'll make some raspberry tea and give you some time alone to think it over."

I rise and wander down the hall, trailing my fingers along the faded flowered wallpaper. In the kitchen, I stare out the window at the early morning light, notice my rumpled, short bowl-cut in the reflection and smooth it down. It's been six years since I chopped my braids off with a hunting knife, in the log cabin in Minnesota, each long rope dropping without a sound on the floor, a symbolic gesture. I was temporarily home from my travels, through with men, and just needed to know who *I* was, separate from their strong, warm bodies. I picked up the braids, a symbol of femaleness, and laid them on the table for Stacy to see.

There was nothing dramatic about our breakup, no café scenes like you see in the movies. Stacy's not an outwardly emotional person. He wasn't then, anyway. He didn't cry or get mad when I told him I was taking the Greyhound to the Peacemakers meeting in Cincinnati and might spend the winter in New Mexico. He accepted it philosophically, the same way he would accept a windstorm that knocked over his bee-hives. He might cuss a little, but then he'd take a few deep breaths, look up at the sun, put the hives back together as best he could, and go on with his work. I carried guilt about the breakup with me like a boulder in my backpack for months.

Abandoning Stacy and Mica was the hardest thing I'd ever done. I wasn't just leaving a man, but the dreams we'd constructed like castles in the air. Mica, for a time, receded to a shining golden sun at twelve noon, reflecting from a pool of water in the bottom of a stone well. He was far away and safe with his father. That year I wandered like a hobo with only a sleeping bag and a few changes of clothes, a traveler through my own great depression.

I spent time in Illinois, Kentucky, and New Mexico, and places in between, Wisconsin, Ohio, and Missouri . . . unsure where to go or how to fill the emptiness. Every few months, I'd bounce back like a rubber ball on one of those thin wooden paddles, but then hit the road again.

Sometimes I took Mica with me. We'd stand together in the grass on the side of a highway, he with his little thumb out, me with a cardboard sign lettered MILWAUKEE, MINNEAPOLIS, or CHICAGO. If a man appealed to me, I slept with him. Then I got sick of it. I was looking for love in all the wrong places. It's a blur when I try to remember.

Fortunately, Colin eventually generated enough energy to give birth to a fledgling community. We rented a run-down farmhouse with a barn that had holes in the roof near Batavia, in southern Ohio. Every few days a new hippie would hike down the road to our temporary headquarters and hang out for a few weeks or a few months.

Mara was there, and Tom, Tristan the Viking, and Kaitlin . . . and some new folk, too many to mention, all of them nonviolent activists. The rooms of the ancient three-story farmhouse filled to the attic with music and politics.

And then one evening, it was late October, I looked out the window into the sunset and there was Stacy with Mica standing in the front yard under a maple that shined the brightest yellow I've ever seen. I ran down the stairs, jumped off the porch, and the three of us fell into each other's arms. The golden maple leaves showered down on us in the slanting light. We were family again and my heart thumped back into my body.

⚘

I glance down at my red plaid flannel work shirt and think how funky I'll look if Grace and Simon decide to go to the hospital. With the palms of both hands, I feel my full breasts. No wet spots, yet. I left a bottle of breast milk with Tom for our baby, but if this labor goes too long, I'll be leaking. I smile, thinking of our auburn-haired three-month-old, Orion, so different from his white-haired older brother, Mica, now seven.

Tom and I got together at the commune after Stacy hooked up with Mara. It was like that back then, musical beds, but we've been together for four years. Orion was born upstairs in the first cabin we built on the ridge, surrounded by our friends from the commune. My labor was shorter this time, but not much. Mica, the little prince, cut his brother's cord by the golden light of the kerosene lamp and we all ate a piece of placenta.

⚘

A Ford truck rumbles up the gravel drive and I wipe my sudsy hands on the back of my jeans. It's Laurel.

From the window, I watch my fellow communard spring out of the neighbor's battered truck. She's as tall as I am, also with short, straight hair, but lighter brown, and she's ten years younger, a dancer with long graceful limbs. In the aftershock of our breakup, Stacy didn't stay long with Mara, but they left friends. He was with a few other partners, but he and Laurel made a commitment two years ago. Like Tom and me, they had a hippie marriage ceremony up on the ridge.

"Hellooo!" The screen door scrapes on the worn green linoleum and Laurel enters. She takes in the kitchen with wide gray eyes, the garbage flowing out of the trashcan, clothes draped over chairs, and the full ashtray on the wooden table. "Where's Grace?"

"Back in the bedroom with Simon. She's in labor, all right, but the baby's only thirty-six weeks' gestation . . . on the edge of preterm. I left them alone to decide what to do. It's a little chancy to stay here, borderline for homebirth, but if we head for hospital now, we could end up delivering in their truck on the way."

"Hey." Simon waves to Laurel as he slouches into the room. He rolls a cigarette and turns to me. "Grace says the contractions are picking up. We're gonna stay home . . . It's a beautiful day, can she go outside?"

"Sure, Simon, but you better stop smoking in the house . . . you know? There's gonna be a kid here in a few hours." The bearded man gives me a sheepish grin and stubs out the cig.

❧

While Laurel sterilizes linen in the oven, readies the kitchen, and makes the birth bed, I brush Grace's long brown hair and tie it back with a blue ribbon, then follow the mother and father-to-be, from a distance, as they stroll around the backyard. I don't need to ask if the contractions are harder. I can tell by the way the woman breathes. And I don't need to give Grace much guidance, either.

Every few minutes she stops, with her eyes closed, sways back and forth, puts her arms around her husband's thin waist and leans into him. He strokes her back and runs his hands down her bottom. They've got a good routine going and I see by the way Simon touches Grace that despite the fact the man doesn't seem like much of a farmer, he's a good lover.

From my seat on a rusted iron bench, under a spreading white oak, I time Grace's contractions on Tom's Timex. I've been delivering babies for two years, but I still don't have a watch of my own. When we moved to West Virginia, the first thing I did was start childbirth classes, again at the local library.

The Roane County Hospital was as restrictive in its obstetrical protocols as St. Mary's and St. Luke's in Duluth, maybe worse, and hippie women, transplants from places like Arizona and New Jersey, New York and California, who had read *Spiritual Midwifery* by Ina May Gaskin, needed my support. Their friends had used midwives and they wanted an unmedicated, natural delivery.

At the time, I'd given birth to Mica and seen two other babies born in the hospital as a labor coach, so I was recruited. I did my first homebirth by accident, when a friend went into labor during a spring snowstorm, and after that I took my well-read copy of *Varney's Midwifery* everywhere.

BLOSSOM

A monarch waltzes across the yard and lands on a drooping daisy. A V of migrating Canada geese flies low over the field, heading south already. It's so peaceful I'm almost dozing, sitting there in the sun, until Grace groans. It's a sound I know well.

"Grace," I call, "I think it's time we go in the house. I want to check your progress. If you aren't close to pushing, we can come back."

"Couldn't she have the baby outside?" Simon asks. "It's warm and she's doing great. There are no neighbors nearby. We could lay a quilt and some pillows on the grass . . ."

Wouldn't that be great to have a baby outside? Like making love outside! For a moment, I'm tempted.

"Nah, Simon. Not this time. Come on. There's more breeze than you realize. We can't take a chance with the baby losing heat." I take Grace's arm and guide her up the steps toward the back door as she looks back at the asters and daisies.

"Ummm!" the mother groans again, grabs a peeling white porch post, gushes amniotic fluid, and waves desperately for her man. Simon rushes forward as Grace drops into a squat.

"No you don't." I pull her up and get her moving again. "No pushing yet. Blow! Let's get you inside and I'll check you." The kitchen is sparkling, dishes put away, trash removed, a jar of wildflowers on the table. Even the window over the sink shines. Laurel runs ahead to open the birth kit.

It doesn't take long. By the time I get Grace back onto the bed, she can't help bearing down. "I've gotta get this thing out of me," she growls, feeling the pressure in her rectum.

"Slow it down, Grace. The baby's right here. Breathe. Show her how, Laurel . . ."

My friend doesn't hesitate. She crawls on the bed, takes Grace's face between her hands, and starts blowing. "Like this," she says. "Hoo, hoo, hoo."

Now all three of them are doing it: "Hoo! Hoo! Hoo!" I pull on my gloves. Laurel hands me the olive oil as I massage the perineum and two pushes later a scrawny baby, with bright red hair, is crying in my hands. The placenta follows with the next push.

"Blossom! It's Blossom!" Grace sobs. Simon wipes his eyes with the back of his hand, but he can't stop crying. He reaches out to touch his daughter and she grips his little finger.

"Here, Simon, strip off your shirt. Your body is the best infant warmer." Laurel lays a very pink baby on the man's chest. I take a warmed flannel blanket, fold it over, and then tuck the quilt around all three. The red-faced infant looks surprised to be here. Her temperature's perfect, 99 degrees, and her respirations are regular.

As Laurel and I retire to give the new family time alone, I throw one arm around my friend's shoulder. The morning sun still shines through the tall goldenrods at the edge of the garden.

Hush little baby, don't say a word . . . Grace's voice floats through the open bedroom window. Simon harmonizes in a reedy tenor. *Papa's gonna buy you a mockingbird.*

Home

The sound of a cat being tortured comes from the bedroom at the far end of our log house, where Rachel is screeching on her new fiddle.

"Shit," Tom whispers, squeezing his eyes shut. He was a music major at Ohio State University before he dropped out and became a draft counselor. He runs his hands over his high cheekbones and sparse beard.

I glance toward the big central room upstairs, where Mica and Orion are sleeping. I'm willing the sounds not to enter their dreams. Mica won't wake, but his little brother, Orion, is more sensitive, easily stimulated, and hard to soothe.

"Rachel . . ." I call, knowing Tom won't say anything. "Do you think you could play a little *quieter?* The kids are sleeping."

"I live here too! When am I *supposed* to practice?"

Ben, upstairs in the far bedroom he shares with Mara, yells down, "Not at night!" I picture his grin, his curly brown hair and twinkling brown eyes. Mara giggles. You can hear everything in this dwelling we call the Long House, and Rachel's been getting on the group's nerves.

"Maybe you could practice in the morning, when Orion and Mica are awake." I try to make peace. Rachel slams her door. Tom and I lock eyes.

It gets harder and harder to live with Rachel, but we cannot ask her to leave. The communal ethics are firm about that. "Everyone is welcome; no one will be turned away." Besides, this farm belongs to a land trust and is hers as much as ours. I let out a long sigh and continue to write in my new green journal. From nineteen members, we are now down to nine, the hard core, seven adults and two children.

Rachel stamps out of her bedroom, a short, stocky, full-breasted woman with pale skin and a shock of red curls. She pulls on her worn sneakers, drags her parka off the hook, and steps outdoors without saying a word. The late autumn wind is no colder than the vibes she trails behind.

"Want some tea?" I ask Tom as I stir up the fire.

"Sure." My husband stretches his lean body, pulls on the boots that he's been oiling, and pushes up his wire-rim glasses. "I better bring in some wood. The temperature's dropping. We might get a frost."

While he's gone, I take up the broom and sweep the golden pine floor, pull out the bench, get the crumbs from under the table, and wash down the wooden counter. I push a knitted draft-stopper against the front door, which opens to the deck that looks downhill into the pine grove, then push another one against the door Rachel slammed, the one we use mostly, that leads to the ridge and the outhouse. I rinse the sink and make sure that the slop bucket's empty.

Rachel bustles back into the house. "Saw Shanti, Fern, and Darla in town today." Her mercurial anger is gone. "They were picking up supplies at the Growing Tree Food Co-op. Shanti's pregnant again. Did you hear? She says she's going to have this one at home. Do you think you'll be there to help her?"

The women she mentions were, until a few years ago, part of our original intentional community. They have moved on and are now living on different farms in the tri-county area.

"I guess. If she wants me." I was Shanti's coach at her first birth, a comedy if there ever was one. Fifteen ragtag hippies and one little blond boy in the Roane County General Hospital waiting room, listening to their comrade scream her way through transition, the part of labor when many women come unglued, and me trying to quiet her. Since then, as a midwife, I've gotten better, learned how to soothe, learned how to listen, learned how to guide.

It startles me to hear my inner voice refer to myself as a *midwife*. When did I decide I was a midwife? For the longest time, I called myself a labor coach or a birth attendant.

Upstairs our three-month-old whimpers. "That's Orion." I immediately cross my arms over my breasts. It doesn't work. The letdown of milk is instantaneous.

"I'll get him," says Rachel.

Ten minutes later the kettle is whistling, my milk dribbles down Orion's little chin, and Rachel sits companionably in the rocking chair next to me. Tom steps inside with a pile of wood and stacks it in the wood box. He's not a big man, but carrying one hundred pounds is effortless for him.

🌱

My turn to go to the outhouse. "Could you change Orion's diapers, Tom? That way he'll be ready to go to sleep when I come back." It's only 9:00 p.m., but without electric lights and TV, we hit the sack early. Then again, carrying water, sawing, and chopping wood, turning over the soil with spades, washing clothes by hand, and tromping up and down this thousand-foot hill makes you ready for bed by dark.

As Stacy and I did in Minnesota, the commune has chosen to avoid power tools in an effort to save nonrenewable fossil fuels. We're devoted to simple, sustainable living and rely on our muscles whenever we can. The difference? Here it's not quite as cold as northern Minnesota, the winter isn't as long, and we are closer to civilization. Also, there are many hands to share the labor, to sing us through hard times and bring in money when we need it.

Outside, the moon, a curved blade, rips through the silver clouds. Though we're only three miles from town, there's no ambient light, no street lamps or neon signs. At night the stars take your breath away, handfuls of stars, buckets of stars, wheelbarrows of stars. There's Orion's Belt and the Seven Sisters just over the stand of pines down the hill, the same as in the North Country.

From the open latrine door, I notice a lantern in the window of Stacy and Laurel's clapboard-sided cabin up the hill. We call it the Little House because it's about the size of our Minnesota log cabin, abandoned now in the North Woods, except for the mice and the squirrels.

We built the Little House, where Tom and I lived when we gave birth to Orion, out of recycled lumber salvaged from a century-old hotel, the first summer we were here. Before that, the hardiest of us slept in the barn and in tents, even when it snowed that first spring, and the rest of us in a little gray house that Shanti rented on Spring Creek Road.

All we had when we came here was two hundred dollars and the muscle of nineteen strong bodies. The light in the window flickers out. Stacy and Laurel must be going to bed.

On the way back to the Long House, I throw back my hood, enjoying the quiet. A barn owl hoots from up on the ridge. I picture the big raptor, high in the treetop, still as a fence post, its yellow eyes blinking.

When I open the door, I smell wood smoke but the kitchen is empty. Only the Coleman, on the hand-built oak table, lights my way. I stand for a moment in the center of the room, looking around.

The stout upright pine log walls are pale yellow, almost cream. A drywall partition at the end closes off Rachel's room. An enlarged photo is tacked near the door, a picture taken that first spring, five years ago, of the group of us in the back of a pickup. I step closer to inspect the faces, radiant with hope, laughing and raising tools in our fists like communist revolutionaries or young farmers on a kibbutz.

I blow out the light and feel my way up the stout two-by-four ladder to the center room. Here, I stop to check that the boys are tucked in. Tom waits for me under the covers in our room. I pull my flannel nightgown on and climb into the nest of his arms.

"Good night, Rachel," I call down.

"'Night, Patsy."

"'Night, Mara," I project to the far bedroom. Though the thick log walls keep out the elements, sound travels inside as through bamboo screens.

"'Night, Patsy." Mara laughs. She gets the joke. We're the TV family on *The Waltons*.

And good night to all the others who were once part of this commune . . . . gone now. Since the war in Vietnam ended, one by one, our friends, no longer needing the strength of solidarity, have drifted away to get real jobs, organize poverty programs, or go back to school. Every time someone puts on his or her backpack and walks away, it's like a tiny sliver of my heart is sliced off.

"'Night, Ben," Tom says, deadpan.

"'Night, Tom," Ben answers in his lower voice. I can feel his sardonic smile.

"'Night, Mica and Orion. 'Night, Stacy and Laurel, asleep in the Little House," I whisper.

"'Night, dancing maples and barn owl. 'Night, stars."

CHAPTER 2

Morning

Morning has broken, like the first morning . . . I set my two buckets of water down carefully, flex my sore hands, and stretch out my arms to greet the world. From here, my view goes on for miles, but I can't see a single dwelling or road, not even smoke from a chimney. We're standing on the roof of Roane County. Where there isn't pasture there are trees, thick forests of yellow poplar, red maple and oak. There's no vehicle noise; no voices but the ones I know.

Rise. Shine. Give God your glory, glory. That's Stacy, from the porch of the Little House, singing his morning song. Rachel scrapes on her fiddle out in the woods where she won't bother anyone. Mara laughs below in the garden as Ben does a rowdy rendition of "Jeremiah Was a Bullfrog."

❦

We found this seventy-five-acre farm by chance, on our first trip into West Virginia. For months, in pairs, we'd been making forays from our temporary headquarters in Batavia, looking for cheap land. On our first trip together, Tom and I, driving Shanti's green Dodge, stumbled onto a long-haired dude with ripped jeans sitting on the curb in Spencer.

"Hey, man." Tom squatted beside him. "We're looking for a cheap farm in the area. Heard of any land for sale?" While I'm sometimes shy, he'll talk to anyone.

"Ask Ira at the Growing Tree." The elfish longhair pointed to a small whole-foods store upstairs in a corner brick building. There, we were shown a handwritten note, in shaky script, on the bulletin board. *For Sale: Seventy-five acres—good hardwood timber and open fields. $7,500. Firm. 927-3008. Sadie Shoepeck.*

After reporting back to our communal center in Batavia, consulting with the rest of the group, and gathering up what little savings the members had, Colin called a friend in Atlanta.

Honey Harriman, Peacemaker, heiress to a cleaning-product fortune, who, like Stacy, didn't believe in inheritance. She wired us the money and the land was ours.

᪄

This morning, the curved green horseshoe ridge is the green of Ireland, so clean and smooth, with the hay cut short by Randall's mower . . . Randall Shoepeck is the previous owner's one-armed forty-five-year-old son. His left arm was torn off in a motor-vehicle accident on a narrow county road when he was a teenager, but he can still work and drive. The whole Shoepeck family has adopted us.

There's Sadie Shoepeck, who sold us the land, the matriarch, a stick of a woman, eighty years old, a timberman's widow since she was fifty. There's Randall the one-armed, and his spouse, Essie, and their almost grown children, Junior and Betty . . . and Randall's older brother, J.K., who lives with his wife, Willene. They all reside along Little Spring Creek at the end of the hollow. This is the way of it all across West Virginia; families living so close they can throw a loaf of bread from one house to the other.

We now see the Shoepecks two or three times a week, but when our spring ran dry that first summer, Randall brought containers of water up the steep hill in his four-wheel-drive truck every evening. I glance back at the well near the barn, where three peeled oak posts make a tripod from which hangs a cylindrical bucket on a rope and a pulley, and remember.

Water Witch

The August day Randall Shoepeck bumped up the hill with old man Booker, the full moon shone in a clear morning sky. A good sign, I thought. At an elevation of one thousand feet above sea level, the chance of hitting water was remote, and we needed all the luck we could find. It was our second spring on the farm. All along the curved ridge, the redbud and dogwood were blooming and the hills beyond were dotted with white wild-cherry blossoms.

Mr. Booker, a water witch recommended by Sadie, was known to be reliable and cheap. Our commune was divided in faith. The men were doubtful, but we women thought, *Why not?* Surely a specialist, no matter how bizarre, would be more successful in discovering water than we would.

☽

Booker, wearing clean black pants pulled up too high, suspenders, and a white button-down shirt, climbs out of the truck, surveys the scene, and then, without a word, begins to stroll back and forth along the open ridge, his divining rod pointing out from his chest.

Some divining rods are made of metal, even bent coat hangers, but Zebidiah Booker's is a forked peach tree branch. Back and forth he marches in the heat through the tall yellow grass, back and forth, without a break, his thin face a mask. Twelve of us silent hippies, varying in our optimism, trail behind. We look like the twelve apostles.

For three hours Booker trolls, and then halts abruptly. We all stop with him. Twenty yards from the barn, which was then our kitchen and community center, the forked stick trembles and points straight to the ground.

"Here," Zeb grunts, his first crusty words since Randall introduced him. "You'll have to bore deep." And he was right. The drilling machine we hired, two weeks later, hit good, clean, cold water at seventy-five feet.

☽

I pick up the five-gallon buckets and trudge on, thinking, *This is ridiculous!* We've *got* to save money to have another well drilled closer to the cabins. At the top of the rise, just before the path turns downhill, I set down my buckets and rest one more time. Before me, the well-worn dirt path leads through the forest, past Stacy and Laurel's Little House and down another narrower wooded ridge to the Long House. Turning, I stare back down into the valley. The sun is just coming over the trees. I hold my arms wide again, palms outward, saluting the morning, saluting those who bear water, saluting the silent, empty sky.

Trillium Stone

Tom pulls me closer and adjusts the quilt over our shoulders.

We're lying naked under the outcrop of sandstone that is our special place, a tiny open cave, down in the woods where the trillium flowers bloom in the spring. Actually they bloom in forests everywhere from Minnesota to Georgia, but here among the rocks you can find them in profusion, large, single, white or occasionally purple-tinted, trumpets. Mara is watching the baby and this is Mica's week to stay with Stacy and Laurel. He has a bed and toys in both houses.

There won't be many more days of Indian summer in which we can escape to make love outside. Fall equinox has come and gone without celebration. Trillium Stone, that's what we call this hideout. Tom gets the joke. "Trillium Stone" was my pen name when I wrote for *The Wild Currents*.

"Hey look." A fuzzy black caterpillar crawls up Tom's wrist. "Sadie Shoepeck says it will be a hard winter. You can tell by the length of the black stripe on the woolly. See here?" He places the two-inch-long black and brown fuzzy larva in my hand. "The bigger the dark area, the colder the season. This one's half black in the midsection. Sadie says we can mark her word, a bad winter coming!"

I let the little caterpillar go into the fallen leaves and snuggle against his body. I've had other lovers, beautiful and exciting men, but this one makes me so happy.

As a young woman I never thought about marriage, except in a negative way, a constraint of the government or a rocky path to divorce. I never aspired to be anyone's wife.

Tom and I had been sleeping together for months when he asked me in a conversational way, "Want to be married?"

"No." I responded. "Why spoil a good thing?"

He continued for six months to ask me again every few weeks. "Want to be married?" The answer was always the same.

And then one day, in the Butterfly Tent, a sloping canvas arrangement on a wooden platform in a field filled with orange butterfly flowers, he asked again.

The poor guy was sick with back pain and fever, probably a kidney infection or maybe a kidney stone. His face was pale and sweaty, the opposite of sexy, kind of pitiful, really. I was putting warm compresses on his back and giving him willow bark tea for the pain. No kneeling in front of me with a diamond ring, just his usual persistent query: "Want to be married?" As sick as he was, his green eyes still twinkled.

"OK." I shrugged. And that was it. No big political shift. No spiritual transformation. It just seemed right.

The next day, at dawn, after Tom's fever broke and he was his old self again, we lay on our stomachs looking out through the tent's mosquito netting at the bright orange flowers and I whispered, "Are we *really* married?"

"Yep."

"Forever?"

He placed his forehead against mine as a pledge. "Always."

ORION

Tom and I were together for two years before we decided to have a baby. We miscarried the first one; I didn't really know it was a girl, but I called her Rainbow. The next one, Orion, stayed with us.

I was two weeks overdue when I went into labor and noticed discharge in my underpants.

Bloody show, I thought—a possible sign of early labor. Word spread on the commune. When the contractions started, everyone kept coming by the Little House to check on me. Stacy, knowing how goal-centered I could get, reminded me with a hug, "Pay attention, not to the clock, but to the goodness of the time."

Finally, Tom and I are alone. We've already fixed up the upstairs of the Little House with all our supplies and Laurel has made up our bed with sterile sheets, so to pass the time we go out on the ridge. The first star appears in the western sky and it gives me courage.

You can do it, the tiny light says. *You can do it.* Tom holds my hand and puts his forehead on mine.

"These contractions are getting hard! Let's move," I tell him. Out along the ridge we march, back and forth, singing John Philip Sousa marching band tunes at the top of our lungs. At the well, we laugh and scream as we pour cold water over each other's heads.

⚘

By midnight, back in the cabin, the contractions are every three minutes. I hold on to Tom and sway in the candlelight. There's nothing outside our room, just him and me and the baby . . . and our portable radio. The music helps. When the channels begin to go off, I frantically demand he search for another one.

I'm staring in Tom's eyes, but I'm looking right through him. He wants to turn me on, rub my breasts like in *Spiritual Midwifery,* but it doesn't feel right and I get snappy.

"Cut it out!"

At 3:30 a.m. he checks my cervix and thinks I'm five centimeters, but if I'd been my own midwife, I would have recognized that earlier note of frustration and anger. *Transition.*

"Let's go see the star again," I command with a note of desperation.

Tom's caught in the riptide now, doing what he can to keep our heads above water. He follows me out into the dark and up to the ridge but the evening star is below the horizon. I'm on my own.

"Let the baby be born," I chant as we march back and forth. "Let the baby be born," Tom chants with me.

Then Laurel comes and we're back in the cabin. "Look at me," she commands, and I focus. I hold on to Tom, grip his back, swaying like a woman in a hurricane tied to a palm tree.

Then, all of a sudden, "Uggghhhhh!" like something primeval.

"Urge to push," I tell Tom, suddenly myself again and all business.

"Blow! Blow!" Laurel gets in my face.

I put my hand inside of me. "The baby's right there!"

"Blow! Blow!" Laurel instructs, but I'm already pushing, slowly at first, like a freight train getting started. When I open my eyes at the end of a contraction, Benny and Mara have appeared and Rachel and Dolly, our midwife friend from Chicago, who we invited just in case we needed her. Stacy sits on the end of the bed holding Mica, whose eyes are like saucers.

"Keep up the good work, buddy." That's Tom as he kneels between my legs and massages my perineum. "You're almost crowning now."

"Ow! Ow!" I complain. "Did you use enough olive oil? Let it come out between contractions, so I won't tear." Between pushes, I'm shouting directions.

"Hi, Mica," I say once, not wanting my little boy to think I'm totally gone.

And then the head is out and the body, still and gray.

"Oh, breathe, baby. Breathe," I whisper. Orion moves his little face and lets out a wail and I know he's OK. Soon he's in my arms, rosy pink. Tom comes up on the bed with me, his face covered with tears. I ask Mica what he thought of the birth and his words knock me over.

"It is like you were fighting for your life, only it wasn't your life. It was the baby's."

Laurel stands back with Stacy. She's crying, too. We are all crying together, every face in the room radiant with light. It's a still, eternal time, a point of God.

CHAPTER 3

Gathering

"Hey. We need some help down here!"

Tom, Mica, and I are in town, taking our turns at the collectively owned Growing Tree Food Co-op, which we purchased from the previous hippie owner, Ira, when he wanted to move back to Syracuse. We bought the stock, took over the lease, and paid for the first month's rent with five hundred bucks, raised from a handful of communes and hippie households.

I'm on my hands and knees in the funky, canary yellow bathroom, scrubbing the floor, when the call from outside, down on the street, interrupts my reflections.

"Hey. *We need some help down here!*" When I stand to peek out the high window, I see Montana, one of the bearded co-op regulars, standing out on the sidewalk next to a big van from the Natural Food Warehouse in Columbus. He's wearing jeans, a tie-dyed T-shirt, and a leather jacket. A leather cord ties back his long hair.

"The truck's here!" Montana yells again, unsure if anyone's heard.

Tom, with Orion on his back in the baby carrier, Mica, and I, with the rest of the customers, thump down the stairs to the sidewalk, then, like a fire brigade, hand sacks of flour, bags of sunflower seeds, buckets of peanut butter, and five-gallon containers of olive oil up the steps to the shop.

At six, we turn out the lights, lock the bright green door, and go out into the dusk, to the Roane County Library a block away. The community room, downstairs, smells of vanilla, garlic, and curry. Seven-year-old Mica and I make big eyes at each other, but it's not time to eat yet and women immediately surround me with babies, many of whom I've delivered.

"No, you don't," I laugh as a chubby cherub reaches for my beartooth amulet and tries to put it in his mouth. His mom takes him back. Then Starlight, Montana's woman, hands me nine-month-old Willow. The golden-haired baby slobbers down my peasant blouse. Her mom's got her dressed up for the party in a blue flowered pinafore. Orion sits on Tom's shoulders, surrounded by a herd of men in jeans and coveralls. Mica scurries under a table accompanied by a flock of shaggy-haired children.

Everyone on the commune has come down from the ridge tonight for this semiannual co-op meeting. Compared to the Armadillo Commune, Circle of the Sun, or the Mudd Farm, we are, with only nine remaining members, a small intentional community, but we are *weighty*. Our commitment to social change, the amount of work we've done organizing the co-op, and the verbal ability of our members, give us import. When the official meeting and discussion of what foods to order is finished, Stacy, Laurel, and Starlight bring out the dinner.

At the far end of the table are bubbling casseroles and big pots of steaming white beans and pintos. Next come the salads and buttery golden cornbread, followed by apple pie, pumpkin pie, and Rachel's gingerbread. Glowing mason jars of homegrown sweet cucumber pickles and pickled beets grace the tables. A pint of our golden honey sits proudly by Tom's home-baked whole-wheat bread. It's a real old-time harvest celebration.

Before we can eat, Montana, compact and blond, the kind of guy who would probably be a Stanford University student president if he weren't a hippie homesteader, asks all of us to hold hands. Without hesitation we reach for each other. Everyone goes quiet as we stand in a circle, close our eyes, and put our love out to the universe. Then Benny, always quick with a joke, breaks the moment. "Rub-a-dub-dub! Thanks for the grub," and the crowd erupts in laughter.

We eat for an hour, go back for seconds, and when every man, woman, and child is full, Montana, Starlight, and Laurel start the singing. *Listen, listen, listen to my heart song. I will never forget you. I will never forsake you. Listen, listen, listen . . .* A banjo and two guitars appear and we move from Sufi songs, to spirituals, to bluegrass, to folk . . .

In the middle of the sing, I get my birth bag and meet with Sue Ellen, a homebirth client, in the kitchen. Sue Ellen, a clear-eyed, wispy twenty-year-old from Delaware, pulls up her baggy thrift-store cashmere men's sweater and shows me her rounding belly.

I have her lie down on the stainless steel kitchen table and do an impromptu OB visit, measuring her fundus and checking the baby's position. I even send her to the bathroom so I can check her urine for protein and glucose. Her boyfriend, Shawn, a former Green Beret, ten years her elder, has also been taking her for prenatal care to the new family doctor in town. "How much weight have you gained?"

"Twenty pounds."

You wouldn't know it by looking at her. There's not an ounce of fat anywhere. I pull my fetoscope out of my bag and check the fetal heartbeat. Her belly and braless breasts are brown; you can tell she runs around on their farm without a shirt, like we all do.

"Can you feel the baby move?"

"Oh, all the time." Sue Ellen smiles. I put my arm around her, help her down from the table, and we go back to the party.

Wearing a long green feather as I fly . . . Everyone is still singing, song after song.

Paul and Silas bound in jail. Had no money for to go their bail . . .

Peace I ask of thee, oh river . . .

Forty or so men and women in harmony . . . until the kids get cranky . . . and our voices give out . . . and again we form a human chain around the room.

Amazing grace . . . Someone starts the closing song and our voices soar up out the high windows into the night. *How sweet the sound* . . .

WILLOW

"What?" Rachel asks. "What's the matter?" Her almost-black eyes snap with concern.

I put down the receiver unable to speak, my throat full of stones. Everyone around the oak table in the Long House stares. The light in the room has dimmed, as if someone turned down the kerosene lamp.

Mara stops serving and her ladle clanks into the soup pot.

"What?" Rachel asks again.

"That was Fern. She called to tell us that Willow, Montana and Starlight's baby, is dead." Mica runs to me and puts his arms around my waist. He knows baby Willow from the Growing Tree. He knows what *dead* means. No one else moves.

Then, all at once, an outburst of voices.

"Fuck!"

"How?"

"No, it can't be!"

I join them at the table, flip my long skirt over the bench and push my soup back. My stomach is sick. Mica crawls up on me and I hold him tight. "It happened a few days after the co-op potluck. Some kind of infection. The baby threw up once, but Montana and Starlight thought she just had an upset stomach, you know, nothing worse." The pea soup grows cold.

"Starlight wiped up the vomit and changed the baby . . . "

Only days ago I'd bounced the cherub-faced infant. Only days ago, I'd held her warm body, in the little blue flowered pinafore, against me at the co-op potluck. Now she's gone. I can't comprehend it. I take a big breath and swallow hard.

"Anyway, Starlight nursed the baby and put her in the crib across the room from their four-poster. Sometime in the night, Willow whimpered twice but went back to sleep and then, close to dawn, just as the sky was getting light, she made a strange noise." I catch Tom and Stacy's eyes. *How many times have our babies stirred and we waited in the dark, hoping they would go back to sleep?*

"When Montana finally got up to light a lantern, he pulled back the covers and found the baby all mottled and blue."

"Like crib death?" Tom asks.

"No, something weird. Spots all over and she wasn't dead yet. More like blotches than a rash and she was hot and lethargic. When her eyes rolled back in her head, they knew something was terribly wrong. Montana got dressed and took off running for the nearest house with a telephone. Because of the mud, their truck was out at the end of the road, over a mile away.

"Fern said it took an hour for the squad to get there and the baby was already dead, but the county coroner feels it wouldn't have mattered. Willow's blood cultures showed a rare type of meningitis. Even if they'd been able to get to the hospital, antibiotics couldn't have saved her."

No one stirs. No one says anything. We're immobilized with shock and sorrow. *If a baby's parents love her and breastfeed her and don't let her swallow buttons or coins, she isn't supposed to die. That's how we think. She isn't supposed to die. If you do what is right and love each other and think good thoughts, bad things don't happen.*

Finally (this is Tom), "Will there be a service?"

"Fern says no." Orion, in his wooden high chair, is banging his spoon on the tray. I pick him up and hold his fragile life against me.

"Montana and Starlight are packing up and leaving for California tomorrow, going out west to be with their families for a while."

There's nothing more to say. Tom stands to push a log in the fire. Rachel begins to scrape plates. No one has finished dinner.

Outside, the first snow begins. Stacy pulls out his Autoharp. *Listen, listen, listen to my heart song. I will never forget you. I will never forsake you.*

The flakes, like gravel, drop straight down. Soon the pine trees are covered, every twig and branch, but there's no dancing in the forest with outstretched arms this night. Willow is dead.

Winter

CHAPTER 4

Healing

"How hot is he?" It's Dr. Dan Schorr on the phone, the hippie physician from the little town of Otto, thirty miles away. "Do you have any Children's Tylenol?"

Orion is sick. His little body clings to me, almost trembles, makes me, too, feel hot and sick. When I try to put him to the breast, he whines and turns his head. His cry is high and pitiful. I remember when Mica and Stacy had the flu on the homestead in Minnesota. Mica wouldn't eat and was listless, but this is worse. *I also remember baby Willow.*

Outside, snow again falls, blows sideways in big thick flakes like scraps of paper. The pines in front of the Long House are already plastered and there's eight inches on the ground from before. Mara, putting up the colored paper chains she and Mica made, watches me over her shoulder. She knows I wouldn't be calling a doctor unless I was really worried. She also knows we have thirty-three dollars in the money jar, not enough to pay for a hospital admission.

"I just took a rectal temperature, it's 104. We don't have any Tylenol, maybe some aspirin."

Dan interrupts. "No aspirin." He has a slight German accent. The practitioner grew up in Connecticut but studied medicine in Frankfurt. He's a Patch Adams sort of doc, practicing out of his farmhouse.

"You don't give aspirin"—*aspireen* is how he says it—"to babies. It could cause Reye's syndrome, but you need to get the fever down somehow. Try bathing him every two hours in tepid water. Take his temperature again between baths and call me if it's still above 101."

"OK . . . OK . . ." I'm writing this down.

"Don't let him get dehydrated or he'll have to go into the hospital for an IV." I give my report to Tom and he tromps through the snow, a quarter mile to the well, for two more buckets of water, then a quarter mile back. I want to ask my husband, "Will our baby die?" but I can't say the words. I want him to tell me I'm being ridiculous. "Don't talk like that, Patsy! Don't think like that."

In the Long House, Mara, Rachel, and I settle down to bathing Orion in a big tin tub. By sunset, Orion's temp is down to 100 degrees, but he's whimpering in a quivery, thin wail and trembling all over. "Shit," Tom says. "What's wrong with him? It looks like pre-seizure activity to me, but what do I know? I've never seen a seizure before."

At seven thirty, when the fever starts to go up again, Tom picks up the phone. "We've got to do something." He dials Dan Schorr.

"Dan? It's Tom Harman. I'm sorry to bother you. The baby's fever went down when we started the baths, but it's back up to 103 and he won't nurse. Do you think we should take him to Roane General Hospital? The snow's a foot deep here and still coming down. We don't have snowshoes, but we could do it." I'm standing next to him with my head on his shoulder, trying to hear what Dan says. Tom tilts the receiver toward me.

"No, don't go to the hospital," our physician friend tells us. "You don't have insurance. You don't need to take the baby out either; the cold might make him worse. I'll come to you."

Two hours later, a call, "Halloooo!" comes from the trees above the cabin and Tom and Dr. Dan, followed by Stacy and Laurel, stomp in. Tom had walked out to Steele Hollow Road to meet Dan and had stopped at the Little House on his way back, to give our friends an update.

On a peg near the door, the family physician hangs his cowboy hat and rough sheepskin jacket. He sets his small black leather valise, the kind Doc Holliday on *Maverick* carried, on the oak table.

❦

Upstairs on our elevated two-by-four bed, Dr. Dan, a balding thirty-five-year old with a dishwater ponytail, begins his examination. Tom, Ben, and Stacy stand at the edge of the kerosene lamplight like the three bearded wise men. Mara sits cross-legged on the blue patchwork quilt, holding Mica. Then Rachel and Laurel, their eyes dark with worry,

creep into the room. No one speaks. Our beautiful baby lies flaccid, his
eyes glazed and vacant, his cheeks red with fever, his temp now back up
to 104. I'm waiting for the blotches. One red spot and we're out of here.
I don't care what Dan says. I'll carry Orion all the way to town through
the snow by myself.

The doc shakes his head, replacing his otoscope and stethoscope in
the black leather bag. "Without blood work I can't be sure, but his tym-
panic membranes look like crap, so I'm betting it's an ear infection. I
brought along some pediatric antibiotics and Tylenol." The doc gets out
a dropper and persistently feeds Orion some syrupy red stuff. There's
no sound in the room but the baby's whimper.

"Maybe we should say a prayer . . . or something . . ." Mara offers.
The group moves spontaneously toward the bed, eager to do anything.
It's not that we all believe the same way, but whatever plea we can
put out to the Great Spirit can only help. For ten minutes we sit in a
tight circle, each person resting a hand on our baby. Mica watches with
round, blue eyes and holds one of his brother's little bare feet. We can't
stop thinking of Willow, how she whimpered in the night and a few
hours later was dead.

By dawn Orion stops trembling. The fever is gone. He's nursing and
pulling my hair. Whether it was prayer or the cherry-flavored penicil-
lin, we'll never know. I favor prayer, love that floats up in the air, does
a slow dance with the stars, and comes down with the cool breath of
heaven.

Winter Solstice

"Fourteen hundred of us were arrested at the last demonstration of the
Clamshell Alliance against nuclear power," Colin rattles on as we pa-
rade through the woods, dressed in parkas, knit caps, and scarves. His
orator's voice rings through the trees. He came with a friend, a young
blond guy from Vermont, for the winter solstice celebration. It's the
first time we've seen him in more than six months.

On the top of the rise, we stand for a moment to admire the sun,
resting over the last row of hills like a Christmas orange, then head

toward the center of the horseshoe-curved ridge where Stacy and Tom have built a bonfire. On this longest night of the year, Anne Margaret, our new neighbor, and her six-year-old son, Joshua, have joined us too. The little boys run on ahead, one stocky and brown, one thin and pale with white wispy hair. We are excited to have another kid around for homeschool. Benny troops along behind, with Orion, bundled up like a mummy.

Colin never wavers in his commitment to nonviolent resistance, but lately I wobble. The loss of Willow, the soft pink baby in the blue flowered dress, has sobered me, made me review my priorities, torn me from the revolutionary barricades down to cold earth.

♈

Anne Margaret sits hunched near the bonfire like a gargoyle, the hood of her wool cape over her head. The lanky hard-faced woman, who recently purchased the adjoining farm, is another Peacemaker that Colin, like the Pied Piper, seduced. Our neighbor has a difficult road ahead, a single mother in rural West Virginia, white with a black child, trying to make a go of it on the land by herself.

I park myself on the log next to her, shoulder to shoulder. "How's it going?" I ask, taking Orion from Benny. Anne Margaret reaches over and touches the baby's cheek with one finger. She rests it there for a second, while Orion gives her a one-toothed grin, then drops her hand back into her lap. The thirty-four-year-old's forehead is perpetually creased.

"I'm OK, but my roof's leaking again; I thought I fixed it."

"Maybe we could come over. Make a workday of it."

"No thanks. I can do it."

I take a deep breath. She's so independent, *never* wants help.

The sun wavers, trembling behind the black silhouettes of trees. We reach for each other's hands. *Thank you for this beautiful world and for the blessings of these friends.* I put my heart out to the universe. *Help me be a good mother, be kind and fearless. And keep us safe. Keep us all, safe.*

I know this is not a reasonable prayer. The world is not safe. Baby Willow was not safe. Baby Willow is dead.

CHAPTER 5

Snow Fight

"So, do you want to go with me?" Mara asks. "We could bum a ride to Highway 50 and then hitch to New England. I'd like to get into some action again but Ben's not into it . . ."

"I don't see how I can. For one thing, I'm still breastfeeding. I'd have to pump milk and throw it away or take Orion with me, and it's so cold; I can't take a chance with him getting sick again . . . For another thing, Alexandra from the co-op is expecting soon. I can't just cut out . . . Hey, no fair!" A clunk of snow whacks me on the side of the face and the cold fluff drifts down my neck.

"Keep me out of it. Anyway, how come no one's helping? Mara and I are shoveling like slaves while you guys kid around! We're not done yet." The day is cold and sunny. Trees clink with ice in the wind and there's seven inches of new white stuff on the ground.

Stacy, Ben, and Tom are chasing each other through the woods, while we women shovel the trail to the latrine. The overgrown boys hide behind trees, aiming snowballs for the head. If it weren't for their pacifist beliefs, they would make good soldiers, tough, disciplined, surprisingly aggressive, able to suffer without complaint, wily, intelligent, and strong.

"Tea time!" Rachel yells from the porch. "Come for tea and muffins." We clomp down to the Long House, stomp our boots, brush snow off our backs, and shake our knit caps. "Whatcha makin'?" asks Ben, eyeing the mess of cut-up plastic tarp all over the floor.

"Sleds," Rachel answers. "One for each of us. After snack, we'll go sledding on the other side of the ridge where there aren't so many trees."

As the shadows of the bare maples and oaks stretch out across the snow, we trudge up the thirty-degree pasture slopes and whiz down on our plastic sleds, again and again. It's like flying.

Ben zooms past. "Race you, Tom!"

These are the good days. There used to be more. I remember when there were nearly two-dozen of us making music in the full moonlight on the top of the ridge that first spring. Mara and I danced naked, leaping and hopping in the moon shadows . . . So many are gone; these last few I hold dear.

The sun is just setting, golden, behind the West Virginia hills when Rachel urges everyone to come back to the Long House for dinner. I watch as Stacy, one arm around Mica and one fist raised in the air in the sign of the revolution, hurtles down the slope one last time. Mica's hood falls back and his white hair blows against Stacy's black beard.

CARLOS

The last time I hitchhiked out of West Virginia was when I went to Austin to apprentice as a midwife over a year ago. It was a balmy spring day, the kind of morning you feel something good will happen. Redbud trees bloomed along the road and pink phlox swayed in the ditches. Our friend Louis had dropped us at the truck stop in Ripley on his way to Charleston to get a shipment of bricks for his kiln.

Lori Moon Dog and I sat drinking tea in a booth with our backpacks stashed on the floor next to us. We were looking for a ride in a semi and had a sign laid before us on the Formica table that said GOING WEST. Mica was at home with Stacy and Tom. Orion was still, as they say, a twinkle in his father's eye.

❧

A truck driver with a gap between his teeth and aviator glasses beckons us over to the counter, where he hunches over a slice of cream pie. "Where you headed?"

"Texas. We'll take anything going west," Lori answers. She's a short, tough grease monkey from Arizona, a longtime friend of Colin's and a part-time resident on the farm.

"Name's Sorlie. I'm goin' straight through to New Mexico." He swipes his face with a paper napkin, grabs both our packs, and carries them out to his sixteen-wheeler. A Polaroid of his wife and daughter rests on the dash, along with a pack of Camels and a roach clip with feathers.

Before we get to Dallas, our driver arranges for another trucker to wait for us at a rest stop. "Got a couple of beavers hitching to Austin. Copy?" he says into his CB. Lori and I can't help it. We know he means hot babes, but we crack each other up by squinting and sticking our front teeth out like cartoon rodents.

I'd learned about the Midwifery Collective, in Austin, a few months before when I attended a homebirth on a farm near Huntington. The mother was a transplant from Texas and introduced me to her friend, Annabelle, a midwife and wiry mother of three. I asked for an opportunity to apprentice with the collective and Annabelle generously offered me a room in her house in exchange for housekeeping duties.

✗

Only one birth from the Austin apprenticeship really sticks with me, though I know there were ten.

Annabelle and Feather, another midwife, and I had been pushing with Rosa, a first-time mother, for hours but nothing was happening. It was starting to remind me of Mica's birth. The father, Diego, a Texas state trooper, chain-smoked in the kitchen.

This was different for me and maybe that's why I remember. In West Virginia, the homebirth community was strictly hippie. In Austin, women who birthed at home were of all walks of life. The fact that the dad was a lawman was strange, too. Since our activist days, cops were the enemy, but Diego seemed like a nice guy.

"Do you think we should call Paul?" Annabelle whispers to Feather.

"He gets out of class by three thirty and should be home by five. That's another half hour . . . I'll leave him a message, but let's keep pushing."

We'd already tried hands and knees, squatting, and every other position, but I help the tired mother into the bathroom again, wondering who the heck Paul is.

☩

Forty minutes later, through the open bedroom window, I catch sight of a tall man with a little ponytail coming down the drive. Turns out, he's Feather's husband. Next thing I know, Paul, dressed in shirt and tie, appears in the bedroom. He nods to Feather and Annabelle.

"Hi, Rosa. You having a pretty hard time?" The young woman, who's now back in bed, nods. "I'm Paul, one of the other Austin midwives." This shocks the pants off me. I thought all midwives were female. It never occurred to me that gender wasn't a qualification. What counts is a practitioner's orientation toward childbirth as a normal physiological event, a profound spiritual passage that has the power to change both men and women.

Paul washes his hands, gloves up, and encourages Rosa to relax. "Can you let your legs go?" She takes a deep breath and complies. I watch the man's face, wondering what he's feeling for during the exam; perhaps the ischial spines, two bony prominences on the inside of the pelvis that are the markers used to determine the descent of the fetal head.

The midwife stares into space, getting his bearings. His brows come together. "The head's low, and you are one hundred percent effaced, but I have to be honest, Rosa, you aren't fully dilated. You're only one centimeter."

One centimeter! *Shit, this is worse than when I was told to push at eight centimeters,* and this time *I'm* one of the people responsible.

The laboring woman wails at this news and Diego takes her hand. Annabelle, Feather, and I stand back against the wall, wishing we could just disappear and wondering how we could have collectively made such a mistake.

"The good news is that your cervix is paper thin. I'm going to loosen things up a bit. This will hurt a little, but after that you can rest. I don't want you to push down, unless you absolutely have to. It will only be a

little while. Your baby's head is in a perfect position." While he talks, I
see that he's doing something with his fingers.

"Ow! Ow! Ow!" That's Rosa.

Instinctively I move to the other side of the bed and take the young
woman's moist hand. "Just blow. It will only take a minute, then you
can rest." I say all this as if I know what's happening.

Paul grins. "Now you're three centimeters! Little secret massage I
do. Soon you'll be five. Diego, take Rosa outside for a walk."

Annabelle and Feather bustle around throwing a blue chenille
robe over Rosa's shoulders and clipping back her long brown hair.
I bring a warm washcloth for her face and while they are gone, follow Paul out to the kitchen, where he pours himself a cup of strong
coffee.

"So, how did you become a midwife?" I ask, feeling like I'm asking a
drag queen how he became a cross-dresser.

Paul turns a chair around, sits down on it backwards, and looks at
his watch. "We used to have a certified nurse-midwife in Austin who
did homebirths. When she left the state, Feather was four months pregnant with our third. There was no way we were going to go to the
hospital after delivering the first two at home, so I'd asked Melanie if
I could accompany her to a few deliveries. The plan was just to learn
what I could, so that I could catch our next kid, but it turned out I had
a knack for it and when Melanie left, I started attending other families'
homebirths too.

"The problem was, I couldn't make it during the day, because I
teach, so I trained Feather and she trained Annabelle . . ." He looks at
his watch again. "Should be soon. How about you? How'd you become
a midwife?"

It pleases me that he calls me a midwife, because I'm still thinking of
myself as a birth attendant. Just as I'm about to tell him my story, the
screen door slams and Feather scurries in with the rest of the entourage.
"Urge to push!" she announces and raises one eyebrow at her husband.
"This time for real!"

Paul and I follow the little group into the bedroom, where Annabelle sets out the birth kit and Feather washes Rosa's bottom. Paul gloves up and checks the woman's cervix.

"The baby's head is right at the introitus and it has hair!" He grins. Everyone cheers but Rosa, who's too busy pushing. She pulls herself into a squat and bears down. This time she means business.

"Hold on there!" Paul laughs. "Give us a chance to get ready." He hands a pair of gloves to me and nudges me over to sit on the bed.

I've already delivered a score of babies, but never in front of a group of experienced midwives, and my hands tremble like new leaves. Here there are no trees to lean on or stars to pray to, so I just take a deep breath and do what I know how to do.

"Oil?" I request, and find my outstretched fingers slicked with warm liquid. I massage the vaginal opening and urge the mother to slow down.

"It's going to burn a little," I tell her. "But I'll hold warm compresses over your perineum to help you stretch. Here, reach down and feel your baby's head." Feather guides the new mother's hand and Rosa's eyes get big.

By this time, I've forgotten my mentors. There's only one thing on my mind, a circle of light around the woman's vagina. The head crowns, slips into my hands, and we all cheer when the baby, before it's born, sneezes. Feather pulls the mother's nightgown up and I settle a crying eight-pounder on her chest.

Paul checks between the baby's legs. "It's a boy!"

"My Carlos!" Rosa holds her husband's eyes.

The baby reaches out his arms.

"Carlos means 'free man,'" Diego explains, and lays his hand on his heart.

CHAPTER 6

Expedition

Three nights ago, a sudden late January storm slammed West Virginia. The wind was so fierce I thought a tree might fall on us. Now eighteen inches of snow covers the trail, drifting almost up to the windows, and we're out of clean diapers.

"We'll either have to carry and heat water to wash them or get into town to the Laundromat," I announce to no one in particular.

We're all sitting around the big oak table for breakfast in the cozy kitchen of the Long House, inhaling the nutty smells of oatmeal slavered in peanut butter and honey. Fire crackles in the woodstove. Tom turns to Stacy, "What do you think?"

Stacy shrugs. "Since the phone is out, there's no way to tell, but the roads must be plowed by now. Then again, we'd have to get to Steele Hollow Road first, and we don't have any snowshoes. I wish I'd brought them from Duluth, but I never thought we'd get snow so deep."

"I'll come too. We've got some dirty clothes." Ben brushes his curly hair from his eyes and hangs his guitar on the wall.

While the men dress for the weather, I load Orion's soiled cloth diapers, red, yellow, and blue with a tie-dyed sunburst design, in a bundle and wrap them in a leftover plastic tarp. We don't use disposable diapers because they aren't biodegradable, but since we're relatively close to town, we've gotten into the habit of using the Laundromat, just down the street from the food co-op.

Rachel jots a list of what we need on the back of a used envelope: cornmeal, cooking oil, lentils, wheat berries. "And get some baking soda too," she instructs as she hands Ben one of her parents' five-dollar bills. "I want to make gingerbread again." I raise my eyebrows when I see the money and catch Mara's eye, wondering how much more the woman has stashed in her bedroom.

Rachel's father, Mr. Levine, owns a string of furniture stores in New Hampshire, and the issue of her money has come up before. Everything we own is in common, and most of us feel we shouldn't accept the privilege of family contributions. People in the third world don't have rich relatives to help them out. How can we say we're trying to live a subsistent life when we accept money from outside?

❊

By sundown it's been eight hours, and the men still aren't home. *There's been plenty of time to get to town and back, even if they had to hike the whole three miles.* Rachel lights the kerosene lamps and arranges them on either end of the table.

I think of going up to the Little House to ask Laurel if we should go look for them, but decide to wait one more hour. Mara sits writing, Rachel sits grinding wheat berries into whole-wheat flour, Mica sits on the window seat doing his reading workbook, and I sit staring into space.

Another blast of wind batters the house and outside the world turns white once more as a new storm takes aim. A chill runs through me and it's not from the cold that comes under the door. Mrs. Shoepeck told me what happened to her younger brother. He was trying to get home from Spencer in a sled with a team of horses when a blizzard hit. This was sixty years ago, before Spring Creek Road was paved. He ran off the trail and his sled tipped over. The horses ran away. They found him the next day, frozen to death in a haystack where he'd taken refuge.

Mara pulls the rocking chair up to the fire and lets out a long sigh.

"Worried about Ben?"

"Yeah, but it's not just that . . . I've been feeling so unsatisfied and low lately." This takes me aback and I don't like it. Mara always seems so optimistic, a person who wakes up smiling.

"Maybe it's a monthly thing."

She cuts me off. "No, I've felt this way all winter. A lack of direction." She sighs again. "I keep thinking I want to start over and reevaluate my life. I don't know anymore what I'm doing here." I pour her a cup of sassafras tea, my heart sinking like a hot stone through the snow. I want to plug my ears like a little kid and yell "Nah! Nah! Nah!" but ever the good friend, I sit down and listen.

"I think of all the people who've left the commune," Mara goes on. "I imagine them organizing food pantries in the South, running kids' camps in the Sierras, or working with the Catholic Workers in New York City. Colin wrote me from jail this week. He's still with the Clam-shell Alliance.

"I actually thought of leaving with him, going back to New England when he was here on winter solstice. At least I'd be contributing some-thing . . ."

I stand and busy myself at the sink, twisting my mouth. It's not just that I fear Mara might leave. Her thoughts mirror my own. Once I was full of moral resolution. I thought that with a community of people to share the work, I'd be able to live simply and at the same time, write, organize women's study groups, deliver babies, and start a free school, but it still takes all our energy just to get by. I'm thinking all this, but don't say it to Mara, afraid of encouraging her negativity; too many have already gone.

I glance over at the black-and-white photograph that hangs by the door. It's never a fight or disagreement that causes people to leave, just a slow erosion. *There goes Brother Lenny back to Cincinnati. There goes Kait-lin and Tall Terry, off to Chicago. Now Shanti leaves to live on her own farm with her lover, Jim. Always walking away. Walking away across the ridge . . .*

Storm of the Century

We wait another half hour to eat dinner, hoping the guys will return, but when Mica complains for the third time that he's hungry and Orion starts crying, we put the cast-iron pot of vegetarian stew, a jar of honey, and plate of golden cornbread on the table. The storm still roars and going out to search for them would be crazy.

"Better say a prayer," Mica, our little prince, says, holding out his small hands to Rachel and Mara. I reach for Orion and close the circle.

We sing our Johnny Appleseed song and Rachel is just filling our bowls when the door flies open and Benny, Tom, Stacy, and Laurel stagger in, the men's beards caked with ice. We all crowd around, help them take off their backpacks, unlace their stiff boots, and bring them dry clothes.

"It's bad," Ben starts out. "Way worse than we thought. Couldn't get the truck started, but it wouldn't have mattered, there's no way we could have made it down Steele Hollow without killing ourselves. Nothing's plowed. The only thing moving was old man McCauley on his horse. We followed his trail, three miles, into town." Mara hastily fills bowls of soup for the guys and they stop for a minute to slurp the hot liquid.

"Half the state is still out of power." Stacy takes up the story. "Most of the telephone lines are down, only the main roads are cleared, Route 33 and County Road 119. It's a major disaster all over the Midwest. The National Guard has been called out in West Virginia, Ohio, Michigan, and Indiana. Twenty people have already died. Now it's starting up again."

Shit! And here we were, cozy as anything, in our snug log cabin.

"Some people are calling it the White Hurricane. The food co-op was closed, no one could get in from his or her farms to unlock the door, but the A&P had power from their generator and we were able to shop."

Tom shakes the snow off the backpack and pulls it over to the table. "Do the honors?" he asks Benny.

"Well," says Benny, rubbing his hands together, with a wink at Mica and flashing his eyes at us all. "Let's see what we have here." Mica crawls up on his lap. "First the staples. Powdered milk, peanut butter, beans, cornmeal, baking soda . . . and eggs!" He surprises everyone because eggs weren't on the list.

"And now with Rachel's generous donation . . ."—he draws this out for effect—"Oranges!" We almost swoon; it's been so long since we've had any fresh fruit besides the apples we stored in the root cellar.

Mica grabs for one, but I tell him, "Later."

"*And* . . ." Mara beats two spoons on the oak table for a drum roll as Benny pulls something from the bottom of the rucksack with a flourish.

"Two pineapples!" We all cheer. "Tom picked these up from behind the store."

"I got them out of the Dumpster. They have a few soft spots but someone must have *just* thrown them out because they weren't frozen." He passes them around and we all take big sniffs of the tropical fruit.

"Party time!" yells Rachel. "I'll make some gingerbread."

"Can I help?" Mica squeals.

Sometimes when there's nothing special to be happy about, except that you have your friends around you and no one's lost in a blizzard, you just have to celebrate. The house already smells like baked goods when Stacy gets out his Autoharp. Ben and I get out our guitars and Tom his string bass. It isn't long until the house rocks with music.

Joy to the world, all the boys and girls! We rattle the storm away with our voices, shake the fury from the blizzard with our clogging feet. I look around at these friends. They are my family and I want to stop life right now, hold it just as it is.

Spring

CHAPTER 7

Fire

Spring equinox. Three gray rainy days have turned into this cold moonless night and still Tom's not home from his new job fixing musical instruments in Athens, Ohio, two hours away. Mara, Ben, and Rachel took off for a week to demonstrate with the Clamshell Alliance in New Hampshire. Laurel, Stacy, and Mica went to visit her family in Philadelphia. The last time I left the farm was for Alexandra Murphy's birth, and that was only for a few hours. I thought at first that I'd arrived there too early, Alexandra seemed so comfortable. We sat around knitting, then abruptly the woman decided to take a bath. I should have known. She'd already had five babies.

Upstairs, I hear her running water. Twenty minutes later she's shouting, "Oh, my God! It's coming!" All I did was support the perineum and hold out my hands. Then we had a party. That was four weeks ago.

✴

By nine, I load the heater stove upstairs in the library, stack more wood to the side, and open the chimney flue halfway.

I brush my teeth, don my flannel nightgown, wool socks, and pink knit cap, check Orion one more time, then crawl into my cold bed. So strange to be out here by myself. I'm not sure it's ever happened before . . .

A few hours later, Orion whimpers and I force myself awake. *This isn't right.* The room's way too hot. Half asleep, I study the situation then pull myself up on one elbow. Through the open door to the library, I see why I'm sweating. The tin chimney pipe, where it joins the stove in the library, is shaking from the force of the internal conflagration. It's a chimney fire! I've seen this before in Minnesota and I've read that creosote buildup in a tin chimney, caused by the condensation of smoke, can burn at 2000 degrees.

Throwing the covers back, I stand at the bedside. My mind jerks wildly from one thought to the next. *I could call the fire department, but even if they knew where we lived there's no road to get in here . . . Should I pour water on the fire or let it burn out? Open the flue or shut it? Any move I make might make things worse, cause the pipe to crash down or the metal stove to rupture.*

I shake my hands in distress. *I don't know what to do, but if I don't do something the roof will catch on fire and the house will burn down.*

That thought gets me moving. First, without waking him, I transport Orion into Mara's room at the opposite end of the house, as far away as I can get him from the red-hot heater stove. Then I fly down the ladder, pull on my boots, and run outside to see if the sparks have caught on the roof yet. If they have, there's no hope.

From the slope above the Long House, I see that the chimney spews gold fireworks, like a Roman candle, but so far the asphalt rolled roofing holds.

Back in the dark kitchen, I find only a half-filled bucket of half-frozen well water. "Damn!" I can hear Orion crying over the roar but I can't help that now. I struggle with the bucket up the ladder. *Calm yourself . . . there's no smoke in the house yet. If you can put the chimney fire out, you'll be OK.*

I glance at the water, suddenly unsure. If I throw it on the stove and the metal cracks, the inferno will spread all over the floor and the house will go up like a tinderbox.

From the junk drawer of my mind comes an image of Rachel making gingerbread and a small golden cardboard box on the table. *Is there any left?* Back down the ladder, I kneel below the kitchen sink. *It must be here somewhere!* I grab what I'm looking for, race back upstairs, wrap a sock over my hand, and rip open the door to the firebox.

Flames leap into the room and I can smell hair burning on my arm but I manage to tear open the box of Arm & Hammer baking soda and spray the white powder over the blaze.

In ten minutes, I'm sitting on the cold wooden floor nursing Orion.

The roar has faded and the tin pipe ticks as the metal cools. I gaze at the stove, wondering how close I came to razing the cabin or cremating the two of us.

For a long time I lie awake in the dark, back in bed, under all our covers, nursing Orion; the vision of the red-hot stovepipe is burned into my retina. The cabin reeks of cold smoke.

Assembly

Rachel clears her throat and pulls her red hair back from her face. "If that's settled, I have more new business." She's sitting straight up at the end of the long oak dining table, wearing a worn green and white Dartmouth College sweatshirt.

Mara keeps minutes at the weekly communal meeting and her head whips up from her notebook. *This isn't on the agenda.* We're already worn out from our two-hour discussion of whether to build a road into the farm so that we can bring supplies into the cabins and have access to emergency services. Currently all we have is a primitive dry-weather trail that we use occasionally to haul in building materials.

The question of a road has come up before and I used to oppose it, but my perspective has changed after the chimney fire. Having a way for a fire engine or an ambulance to get into the cabins might someday be critical. And I need to be able to get out if one of my mothers, like Alexandra, goes into labor in a hurry.

In the consensus model of decision making, those willing to argue their point for the longest win. Granted, we avoid the tyranny of the majority over the minority when we make group decisions, but to get everyone in agreement takes hours, sometimes weeks, of meetings. That's why our commune, after seven years, is still called, by other hippies and even sometimes by us, the No Name Farm. We can never agree on a name we all like.

It's the first week of April and Tom squirms in his seat, eager to get out in the fields, haul water, clean the outhouse, *anything* but continue the drawn-out discussions. Both doors to the kitchen are open and the smell of earth and growing things wafts through the room. Rachel's timing is bad. We were just about to end the meeting.

"Shit." Benny throws a wooden spoon across the kitchen. It hits the wall and rattles on the floor. I tighten my jaw. Ben has a temper and this is not the first time we've seen it. The whole group is frustrated.

Rachel stubbornly continues. "My parents have given me some money and I want to build my own cabin." We are shocked. All the dwellings on the farm are so far communal. No one responds.

The persistent woman holds out a piece of lined paper. "I've picked out a site, down in the woods where the wild turkeys gather, and I've prepared a plan. I'm hoping you all will help me." Still no one speaks; we just stare at the hand-drawn diagram dangling from her fingers.

"I'd like to be done by August."

Stacy takes the plan and gazes at it numbly. Ben stares over Stacy's shoulder. Mica breaks the deadlock. He looks up from one of the sheets of numbers that he's continually working on. He chews on his pencil and his blue eyes find Rachel's. "I'll help." A child's opinion is considered as important, on our commune, as an adult's.

By the time we all agree to provide the considerable labor to construct Rachel's dwelling, we're too burnt out to consider the ramifications of a private cabin on communal land and we rush through the doorway to escape the net of our words. It's not just *this* meeting we are fleeing, but *all* the meetings we've endured for the last five years. We need to get out in the sunshine, where the wind can sweep through our minds.

✻

For an hour, there's no sound but the turning of soil, the shuffling of feet, and the crows cawing from the top of the pine trees. Like peasants in a Van Gogh painting, we bend low over our tasks. Across the green hills, the tops of the maples are just turning rose and the dogwood flowers are opening.

Laurel takes off her shirt and her small brown breasts wag as she hoes. Mara throws down her shovel and does a do-si-do with Mica, her ponytail bouncing.

People of the fields, people of the valleys . . . All over earth we toil, Stacy sings.

Strong hearts and hands, tending the land . . . We all join in . . . This is the joy of communal living, the singing, the working together, not the meetings, the never-ending meetings. Ben points out a red fox at the edge of the woods, then we all go back to our labor, the good sun warming our backs.

CHAPTER 8

Unexpected

I'm sitting down near the little creek in the ravine below the Long House working on a song I've been writing. "I have been lost before, and come into these woods to lay my body down." The sun shines down through the new leaves, but there is little joy in me and I don't know what's wrong. "And you have taken me in arms of light and sung to me—rocked me gentle in the tops of trees."

On my way back up the hill, my path crosses Mara's. She stands with her chin up, her wavy blond hair tied back with a blue bandana. "Hey. I've been looking for you. I have something to tell you."

I knew it. Now Mara is leaving. She's been talking about her wonderful week with the Clamshell Alliance ever since she got back . . . I feel deceived; as if I'd been seduced to West Virginia by these beautiful people and now they're all abandoning me. I stare up at the treetops, don't even meet my friend's eyes. *Come on, get it over with, just cut out my heart.*

Mara clears her throat. "I didn't want to say anything until I was sure . . . but . . ." She gives me a shy smile. "Benny and I are pregnant."

"Mara!" I instinctively throw my arms around her, and then pull back to look at her. Her oval face is pink, but it could be embarrassment. "I guess I should ask. Are you *happy* about this? Is this what you wanted?"

"Well, it's not what we'd *planned,* but it's OK. Ben's thrilled. And I am, too. He figured out I was expecting before I did." She rests her hand on her still-flat lower abdomen. "I honestly haven't been sick or anything. I'm a little tired maybe, but that's all. I've missed three periods. I guess I'm due in the fall."

In my mind I run over the women who are due. Sue Ellen is expecting any day now. The Seventh-Day Adventist woman Laurel and I met at the co-op is due in a month, and now Mara.

I had expected the worst, my best friend leaving, but new life is burst-

ing out everywhere. We walk toward the house, arms around each
other. The creek gurgles along the bottom of the hollow. Dogwood
blossoms float like small white clouds on unseen branches up on the
ridge, and Mara isn't going anywhere.

Night Ride

The phone rings insistently into the dark. "Uhhhhhhh," I groan. By the
alarm clock it's 2:00 a.m. I stumble down to the kitchen and stub my toe
on a piece of firewood that's been left near the stove. "Hello."

It's Shawn, our friend from the food co-op, the former Green Beret
who always wears a pair of white Fruit of the Loom underpants like a
cap over his Mohawk. When you've lived through the madness of Vietnam, it probably doesn't matter how crazy you look.

"Hi, Shawn, what's up?" I just saw him twelve hours ago when he
brought Sue Ellen to the farm for a prenatal checkup.

"Not much. What's up with you?" I know the call has to be
about Sue, but I wait for Shawn to come to the point. The man is
wound a little too tight, like a grenade that could go off if you just
brush the pin. You don't want to push him. "My woman's in labor,"
he announces in a voice that sounds like gravel on the bottom of a
miner's pan.

I ask him the usual questions: "When did contractions start?" "How
close are they now?"

"Her contractions are every five minutes and her water bag
popped. The trouble is we're not at home," Shawn explains. "When
Sue Ellen started leaking we stopped at our neighbor's house. We
thought it was pee at first. Can you come, Patsy? Can you come right
away?"

I run my hands through my short, straight hair. *Shit.* Laurel, Rachel,
and Mica are in Charleston at a folk dance festival. Tom is away again
in Athens. Benny hitched to Cincinnati for a Peacemakers meeting. I
don't even know if I can get the jeep started. "OK. OK . . . How far
away are you?"

"Three miles out Tanner's Run at Sam Trout's place. It's a little white house just before you turn onto Boggs Hollow. There's a big red barn on the side."

"I'll be there as quick as I can."

Mara's awake now and has joined me in the dark kitchen. I hang up the phone as she lights the kerosene lamp.

"What's up?"

"That was Shawn. Sue Ellen's in labor. They were just here this morning for a prenatal visit, but her amniotic sac broke on the way home. I gotta get going. Sounds serious; she could be five or six centimeters. Can you take care of Orion? I'll ask Stacy to drive me. He's good friends with Shawn and he's been to their farm."

☿

Thirty minutes later, my ex-lover and I are bouncing along Tanner's Run in our 1950 Jeep pickup, looking for the turn to Boggs Hollow.

The fog is so thick you could spoon it like soup. On the hilltops it clears. In the bottoms we smother. Back and forth we go, through mist and then stars. Windows open, craning our heads, we slow as we approach the next intersection. It's a moonless night, pitch dark. A silent farmhouse squats at the mouth of a hollow where a creek runs under a bridge.

"This is it," Stacy says, throwing gravel as he swings into a long drive between four towering maples. The house is lighted like a Chinese lantern and there's a shadow of a three-story structure to the left that must be the barn. I detect the sweet smell of cow manure and hay.

☿

A thin man with a long gray beard who looks like a guitarist from the band ZZ Top cracks the door open. "Yeah?" he asks suspiciously. For a minute I think we've got the wrong house. Rock-and-roll music blares into the dark.

"I'm Patsy, the midwife, and this is Stacy. Are Sue Ellen and Shawn here?"

"Well, it's about time!" The old guy throws the door wide and the kitchen light and the voice of Meat Loaf spills out at our feet. "Get on *in* here. I thought I might have to deliver this baby myself! How you doin'?" He sticks out his hand to Stacy. I move on past him into the kitchen and set my birth bag on the Formica table, taking in the view. The small room with green striped wallpaper smells like fried onions and cigarettes, but it's tidy.

"They're in the back," Sam indicates with a jerk of his thumb.

While the men discuss the state of the weather, I pick my way through a darkened living room, past stacks of cardboard boxes and piles of folded clothes. A small silenced TV in the corner illuminates my way, and from somewhere Bob Marley informs me in a reggae beat that *"everything's gonna be all right, everything's gonna be all right."*

COYOTE

At the end of a narrow hall, I hear moaning and there find Sue curled on her side wearing nothing but a green plaid flannel work shirt. I'm on alert now. No self-indulgent thoughts about the dwindling commune. That's what I love about attending births, there's no room for mistakes, no place for spacing out. I notice a streak of bloody show on Sue Ellen's thigh. Her long blond hair is neatly braided down her back, her face pink and shining with sweat. Shawn sits at the bedside wearing a black Grateful Dead T-shirt and, as usual, the Fruit of the Loom underpants on his head.

"Take a sip of water," he orders. There's a tattoo of a snake curled around his huge bicep. The young woman takes a cleansing breath, lets out her air, and tips her head back as her man gently holds a mason jar to her mouth.

"They're really *hard,* Patsy. I hope it's not much longer. I don't know if I can make it."

"You're doing great," I tell Sue Ellen, opening my bag and pulling out my fetoscope.

"Yeah, you're doing fine, honey." That's Shawn.

It takes a minute to find the baby's heartbeat and I'm surprised when I locate the sound just above the belly button, not down by the pubic bone where I'd found it this morning. I listen through a contraction and for a full minute afterward . . . one hundred and forty beats per minute with a good acceleration. "Perfect," I tell Sue Ellen and Shawn. "The baby's in great shape. Now I want to check you to see if we have time to get you back to your house."

I pull out a pair of sterile gloves and ask Sue Ellen to roll on her back. Contractions are coming on top of each other, and the young woman doesn't say much, just breathes and does what I tell her. Stacy slides into the room behind me. "Hey, man." He and Shawn grip each other's hands.

With two gloved fingers under the sheet, I follow the vagina up to the cervix. My eyes widen. Seven centimeters and fully effaced already! *We're not going anywhere.* In fact, we'll have to set up right now. I glance around the room. There's an old maple bureau I can lay my birth stuff on. I begin barking orders to the men. "We don't have much time. This baby's coming. Shawn, can you get some of the clutter cleared off the dresser? Stacy, help take everything that might be in the way into the living room."

"I got to push!" Sue Ellen groans, grabbing onto the sleeve of my hooded sweatshirt.

"No, too early!" I command. "Do like this." I puff out my cheeks like I'm blowing out candles, and then my eyes go round. My fingers are still in Sue Ellen's vagina as her cervix opens to eight.

But something's not right. There's a fissure down the middle of the baby's head. I shudder, picturing a deformed child, and then pull myself together. Fetal heartbeat high on the abdomen? Soft cleft in the presenting part? It's not a fracture down the middle of the infant's soft skull, but the baby's *butt crack* I'm feeling!

Now my mind goes into overdrive. I've never delivered a breech before, never even seen a breech delivery in a childbirth movie. The books say there are so many things that could go wrong. The cord could be compressed as the body comes out. The arms could extend and get jammed between the fetal head and the pubic bone. The buttocks could come out, but the head, the larger part, get stuck.

"Shawn . . . Stacy . . . hold up. We got trouble."

Sue Ellen starts to freak. "What? What's wrong?" She looks up at Shawn, wild eyed.

"The baby's fine. No problem there. Good fetal heartbeat without deceleration. But he or she is coming out breech . . . upside down . . . bottom first. I thought the head was presenting when I checked you earlier, and apparently so did Dr. Farr, but your cervix was only a fingertip dilated and we must have been wrong or maybe the baby flipped.

"The point is, things aren't normal. I've never delivered a breech before and it's more dangerous. I'd say we have to go to the hospital right now, but the hospital's an hour away. I'm afraid you'll give birth before we can get there and I don't want to deliver my first breech in a car." I pause. Sue Ellen gives me a fierce look. "I can do it," she says, and I believe her.

"I need a moment," I tell Stacy, squeezing his familiar, strong hand. "Can you lay everything in my birth bag on the dresser? I guess we're staying here . . . and don't let Sue Ellen push."

⚘

It's a warm night outside in Sam Trout's side yard and I find a tree to lean on. The vision of the breech baby that died at Tolstoy Farm pursues me and I need strength for whatever happens tonight. With my arms stretched around a great silver maple and my cheek against the smooth bark, I whisper, "Great Spirit, steady these shaking hands. Help get us through this. Protect Sue Ellen and her baby. Be my guide." My whole body is pressed against this huge living being and when I feel the tree breathe and the leaves rustle above, I'm no longer afraid.

"Miss?" Sam Trout shouts into the dark, his head poking out the kitchen door. "Miss, Patsy. They're callin' for you." I trot back to the house, wondering if I'd been seen hugging the maple. Not exactly a confidence builder, to see the midwife talking to a tree.

In the bedroom, Shawn and Stacy are holding Sue Ellen up. She has her legs open and is instinctively bearing down. The chick knows what she's doing and a tiny butt cheek already shows. *Holy shit!*

"Sorry," Shawn says. "We told her not to push, but she says she has to."

Stacy, always calm in a crisis, has placed my sterile scissors, olive oil, two hemostats, gauze, and cord clamp on a sterile towel on the dresser. On the bed, I spread open a copy of *Varney's Midwifery* to the section on breech births, then glove up and pour olive oil over the thinning perineum.

Sometimes a breech baby will poop in your hand; black gummy stuff called meconium, but Sue Ellen's infant is too refined. Bob Marley sings in the background, *"No woman, no cry. No woman, no cry."*

Shawn's face is white. He's removed his Fruit of the Loom cap and his Mohawk droops to one side. Stacy's eyes are pinned to the presenting part. Sam Trout leans against the doorway, as relaxed as if he's observing a Jersey cow give birth in his barn. I glance again at the illustrations in the medical volume.

Every two minutes, Sue Ellen pulls her legs back, grits her teeth, and with great courage bears down. Stacy wipes the perspiration from her face with a cool rag. Shawn takes the young woman's hand between contractions and presses it to his lips.

With each push, more of the bullet-shaped body appears. I could check the fetal heartbeat with my fetoscope, but what would that prove? If the rate begins to drop, we can't get to the hospital in time for a C-section, and with a breech you can't pull or you'll extend the arms.

"It's up to you now, Sue Ellen! You're almost done. I can feel the cord pulsing, so I know the baby's getting enough oxygen. And she's got her arms at her sides where they belong." I say all this like I know what I'm doing, but it is only the pictures in *Varney's* that reassure.

"Towel," I say to Stacy. If I had time to think about it, I'd be amazed at my daring.

Imitating the directions in the text, I wrap the fabric around the baby's wet hips and lift up. With my other hand, I press my fingertips into Sue Ellen's lower abdomen, cup the baby's head through her flesh and keep the skull flexed.

"This is it, Sue Ellen, everything's out but the head. Push like you mean it, and if you run out of air, grab some more and go down again.

Push until I tell you to stop." The mother pulls back her legs one more time and puts her chin on her chest. Shawn and Stacy, grim-faced, help her sit up. We all bear down, willing this baby to be born. It occurs to me that if we needed to we could lift the whole farmhouse.

The infant's body is out, drooped over my forearm, and slowly, gently, the head delivers, first the nape of the neck, then the ears, and finally, the soft wet black hair. No episiotomy. No lacerations. I let the whole baby fall into my lap, pink and already crying. *Bow down,* I think. *Bow down and sing the praises of the small, the weak, the miraculous.*

We all cry, even Shawn, the hardened, half-crazy Vietnam vet with the Fruit of the Loom underpants now back on his head. "Coyote," he whispers. "Wise little Coyote."

Outside the bedroom window, the undersides of the new green maple leaves reflect the rising sun, and Marley now sings, *"Everything's gonna be all right."* Over and over, *"Everything's gonna be all right."*

CHAPTER 9

Mope

I am sitting with my chin in my hand, feeding Orion oatmeal and staring out the window at the lush green forest. I'm in a mood today, and
I can't tell if it's PMS or something else. Despite the beauty outside,
there's no joy.

The screen door slams and Mara swaggers in wearing her work
clothes, black polyester slacks and a baby blue sweater. She looks like a
secretary on *The Mary Tyler Moore Show,* has a big grin on her face, and
slaps the *Roane County Times Record* on the table.

"What?"

"I found you a job."

"Me?"

"Yeah, *you!* For weeks you've been moping around, letting out these
long mournful sighs. I was thinking if you got off the farm more, it
would do you good. You're too isolated. I enjoy working at the eye doctor's office a few days a week and Rachel really likes taking care of the
old people at the nursing home . . . You need to get out more."

I stare at the folded weekly newspaper and then give Orion another
spoonful. Since Mara announced she was pregnant, she's been way too
spunky.

"Who says I've been moping? I get out now and then; once a week
to the food co-op and occasionally to do a homebirth or make a home
visit. Besides, who would take care of Mica and Orion?" I shoot her an
irritated look but can't help asking, "What's the job, anyway?"

"Oh come on! There are seven of us. I think we can cover child care!"
Mara picks up the newspaper and reads the advertisement that she's
circled in red. "'Outreach Worker wanted to make home visits and
teach sewing, nutrition, and budgeting. Some college required. Must

145

have own transportation' . . . I already called Community Action; the position is still open and Mrs. Hatcher sounds interested."

"Who's Mrs. Hatcher? Anyway, I don't know anything about budgeting. I never had enough money to budget . . ." I think this is funny, but Mara doesn't laugh. She's on a mission.

"You know Mrs. Hatcher! She used to work at the library when you taught childbirth classes and volunteered as Story Lady to read to the little kids."

"Sounds like you've got it all worked out . . . only one thing. *Vehicle.* All we have is the old jeep truck and it's in bad shape."

Mara is blowing my mind. Though I've resented being stuck on the farm while everyone trots off to work, meetings, or demonstrations, I hadn't considered getting a job, not since I got pregnant with Orion, anyway. I'm vacillating somewhere between irritation and interest.

"Well, I've figured out the transportation too. I saw Sara and Fred Meretti at the co-op and was telling them about the position. When Sara's grandmother died, they inherited her new car and they want to give us their old Volvo."

"Give it to us? Why would they do that? They're good friends and all, but *give* it to us? Does it run?"

Mara laughs. "Yeah, it runs." My cynicism doesn't deter her.

Sara and Fred are Peacemakers who live a few counties over. I was with Sara at the hospital for her second delivery. I smile when I think of her yelling at the new nurse, "You better quit diddling around and get the goddamn doctor!" Sara never swore, so she was obviously in transition. I haven't seen the Merettis since the co-op potluck last fall.

"You were Sara's coach when they had their baby girl! They want to give something back."

Orion is sitting in front of me in his wooden high chair, his mouth open like a baby bird, and I remember to shovel in another spoonful of mush. Mara wipes the dribble off his chin with a dishtowel.

My friend's observation is right on; lately I have felt lonely, resenting my place as keeper of the home fires. I rise to put the bowl in the sink and nudge Mara out of the way. She shoulders me back and we stand for a minute in the middle of the kitchen, pushing against each other like two lady wrestlers.

"You got it all figured out, huh?" I grit my teeth and meet her eyes.

"Yep." I'm bigger than she is, though she's just as sassy.

"OK. OK. I'll check it out. For sure we could use the money." I give her an extra strong push then remember she's pregnant and ease up on the wrestling.

Ghost

Cursing myself for my foolishness, I toss my well-worn paperback copy of *Varney's Midwifery* back on the bed. If only I hadn't been stupid and tried to pull that log out of the woods single-handedly, this wouldn't have happened. I was so determined to get a road built into the farm that when the group finally agreed, I *had* to make it happen. My zeal, as we cut trees to widen the trail, outmeasured my strength.

Now here I lie, supine, unable to do anything but breastfeed and tend the baby. Thank goodness Mrs. Hatcher agreed to hold my job. The door downstairs bangs open.

"Mara," I call. "That you?" There's no answer. Then heavy feet clump up the ladder. With each step there's a groan. I think of a bear, but know that's silly. "Tom?" Still no reply. "Hello?" I call out. *Why won't he answer?*

The next thing I know, Tom staggers into the room and collapses on the floor, holding his knee. "Oh, fuck!" he cries. "Shit!" I've never heard Tom go on like this. Ignoring my own back pain, I slide off the bed.

"Didn't you hear me shouting for help?" I shake my head no, shocked by the look of him. "I've been calling and calling," he moans. "Everyone else on the farm is off somewhere."

"You know I couldn't hear. I would have come somehow." I kneel over his injury and try to pull up his pant leg. "What happened?"

He winces. "Fuck! Stop for a minute. I was up on the ladder, almost done shingling Rachel's roof, right at the edge, when a rung broke through and I fell two stories, crashed on the lumber pile below. I finally realized you'd never hear me and scooted along the path on my butt.

Fuck! It hurts so bad, I'm afraid something's broken." His skin is pale, sweaty and cold.

From Boy Scouts, Tom knows how to make a secure splint, and by the time he's done he's pretty sure his leg's not fractured. Though it hurts and takes a good while, he's up on the bed by sunset. He lies beside me, flat on his back, like a man in a coffin, arms at his sides.

Outside the window screen, the evening birds warble in the green summer light. I look down at the scraped-off skin, the purple bruise and swelling. "When you came in, you looked like you'd seen a ghost."

"I did. The ghost of myself, lying dead on the woodpile with a broken neck."

I'm silent, imagining Stacy and Laurel coming to the cabin after finding Tom's lifeless body. I see by their faces that something is wrong. They gather me in. Stacy tells me the news as gently as possible, that my husband, my lover, my best friend is dead. Dead as in gone forever, *as in never going to sing with me again, never going to make love with me again or argue with me or comfort me or play with our boys.*

"I almost bought it, Patsy. We must be doing something wrong." He turns and buries his head in my side, sobs without noise, his whole body shaking.

I've seen tears in my lover's eyes many times, tears of joy, but this is the first time I've seen him cry in earnest. I pat his back and stare out the window. "It's OK, Tom. You're OK now," I whisper. "You're safe now."

Summer

CHAPTER 10

Wider

"Mrs. Utt?" I peer through the rusty screen door into the shadowy interior of this rough, unpainted, wood-sided dwelling. A woman sings along with Willie Nelson on the radio toward the back. She mimics Dolly Parton and doesn't sound half-bad.

This is my first week employed by Roane County Community Action, going to the homes of the poor, teaching sewing, nutrition, and budgeting. Though it's only part-time, a component of the War on Poverty, I'm grateful for the work. We need the money, and it gets me off the farm for a few days a week. Instead of worrying about the commune, I think about the women I visit. The world has grown wider. Mara was right. I'm happier now; find myself singing more, laughing more.

I'm also grateful for the ten-year-old Volvo that our friends the Merettis gave us. I glance over my shoulder at the sturdy faded blue vehicle, parked just on the other side of the creek next to the swinging bridge. Without it, I couldn't have taken this job.

"Mrs. Utt!" I yell louder, pounding on the warped brown doorframe. She'd better be expecting me after I risked life and limb crossing the waterway on that wobbly wood-and-cable contraption.

I hear the slap, slap, slap of flip-flops. "Yeah, I'm comin'. If ya selling somethin', I can't afford it. If ya need a phone, I ain't got one. If ya asking directions, you're mighty lost." A narrow pixie face with a cigarette in the corner of her mouth peers through the screen. Etta Utt, a mother of four, is a lot younger than I expected, mid-twenties, dressed in tight blue stained polyester pants and a striped purple tee.

"I'm Patsy Harman, Mrs. Utt, the home aide from Community Action. Mrs. Hatcher, the director, told me she'd asked if I could visit."

The woman glances at the rooster clock on top of the TV. "Oh, gosh.

I plum forgot. Come on in." She pulls the screen open and waves me in with one hand. The wooden doorframe drags across a curved scar in the bare pine floor.

I check out the living room as I follow her through: baskets of folded clean laundry on a torn imitation-leather sofa that's covered with magic marker scrawls, dust balls in the corners, a jar of daisies in the center of a coffee table propped up with a concrete block.

My hostess and, hopefully, soon to be client, escorts me to the kitchen, where she's been cutting up carrots for stew. I use the opportunity to pull out some healthy recipes I've mimeographed on bright yellow paper. "The application you filled out for the program says you have five kids. Is it OK if I call you Etta? You can call me Patsy."

"Suit yourself." She settles on one of the unmatched wooden chairs at the long rectangular yellow table. I sit down, too.

"Mind if I ask, boys or girls?"

"Two boys, the twins. The rest is girls." Etta scratches a wooden match twice on the bottom of the chair and inhales another unfiltered Camel. In the light through the window over the sink, her small face with high cheekbones is more lined than I thought. She could be thirty, even thirty-five. I pull out some fabric and together we clean off the table.

Tiny Mrs. Utt tells me about her children as we lay out the Singer pattern for a simple blouse on the kitchen table. In the few visits I've made, I've discovered that my welcome in these impoverished homes is based on my having something tangible to offer. What insures my acceptance is not my recipes, or tips about making the most of one's money, but the colorful cloth I bring. New flowered gingham is the ticket that gets me through the door.

"The twin boys are in seventh grade, then one of the girls is in fourth, and the other in third," Etta explains.

"You were popping out babies every few years weren't you?" Birth stories always interest me.

"Got knocked up nearly every twelve months. Lost a few too. Been pregnant ten times. Besides the ones living, I had three that didn't take and one that came too early. That was the worst. Poor little thing. The last one . . . He weighed just two and a half pounds. Didn't seem like they tried very hard to save him. I heard Doc Carson tell a nurse that I already had too many damn babies. Wasn't his business how many kids I had!

"They just took his little body away. I never even got to hold him . . . We wanted five or six kids. Sparky had a good job at the rubber plant, before he threw his back out. The doctor put me to sleep and cut out my tubes."

"Sterilized you?"

"Yeah."

"They can't just sterilize a woman against her will." This pierces me like a sewing needle stabbed through the thumb. Not just the injustice but the assault on the woman's body.

"They *can* and they *did*. Afterward, Dr. Carson told me I was bleeding too much and it would be a danger to have more children." She barks a short laugh and exhales smoke through her nose. "I wasn't bleeding that much. I'd had babies before. He thought I was dumb."

I take a long breath and show Etta how to pin the front of the golden daisy print smock to the back, placing the pins so she can stitch over them.

I don't know what to think about Etta's physician. In her limited circumstances, five babies seem like too many, but it wasn't for Dr. Carson to decide. "I'm sorry that happened to you," I say softly. "Losing the baby and the doctor sterilizing you . . ."

"It's OK," Etta answers through the pins in her mouth. The Camel smolders on the edge of the table. "I'm grateful for what I got, my other kids and my husband, Sparky. He treats me real good."

Two hours later I stand at the front door with my hand on the screen and make plans to see my new client the following week. "Oh wait!" The little mother flies back to the kitchen. "I plum forgot. I fixed you a poke with a few cookies and soda."

As I shuffle back over the swinging bridge to the Volvo, careful to step over the missing boards, I can still see Etta leaning against the porch post and I raise my hand in salute. She waves back and pushes a strand of her brown hair behind her ear. Wild pink sweet peas grow on the riverbank. I remember it's summer solstice today and throw a handful of blossoms into the water.

Betrayed

"You mean leave the farm?" My voice is high, filled with tears, but I try to hide them. When I look up, the sun has dropped behind the court-house and the street is in shadow. What I've feared for months has finally happened.

The three of us, Mara, Rachel, and I, are waiting, on the public bench across from the food co-op, for a ride back to the farm with Randall Shoepeck. This is the first mention Mara has made of her plan to move to town.

"For good? Both of you?" I'd been lulled into trusting her and thought that now that she was pregnant, she'd stay put. I'm almost choking and I'm furious too, but I can't say this.

"Benny's job wouldn't start for a month. He just got the offer last week. I didn't want to say anything until I was sure. The pay will be good and the Spencer State Hospital will even pick up his tuition if he wants to go back to school. We'll get health insurance and they're giving us a house on the grounds, rent-free. We just can't pass it up. Besides, I can be more involved with the local community."

Mara has just told us that Ben is starting work as manager of land-scaping at the huge old brick monolith on the edge of town, a mental hospital, one of the largest employers in the county. Randall Shoepeck works there and put in a good word for him. I bristle when she says she'll be more involved with the community. What about *our* commu-nity? What about the farm?

Mara continues to try for my support. "It's a four-bedroom two-story house and can be a home away from home for all of us," she goes on. I'm barely listening. "It's a great deal. We'll have indoor plumbing and electricity. Everyone can come to town and take showers and do laun-dry. And Benny will get four hundred dollars a month. We'll be able to save money to get the new road graveled, maybe even convince Anne Margaret to sell us permanent access."

"But you won't be with us when you have the baby. What are you going to do? Have it in the hospital?" I throw this out in a mean way, but I can't help it.

"You'll still help me have him in our new home, won't you?"

"Yeah . . . I guess . . . but are we supposed to be happy?"

Rachel, on the other end of the bench, hasn't said a word. The red-haired woman lets out a heavy sigh, stands, and strolls toward the Growing Tree as if nothing's happened, as if she's not concerned, not involved. Since we started building her little chateau, maybe she doesn't care anymore. Maybe she's already given up on the commune. The Growing Tree's bright green door slams behind her.

"Well, I hope you'll enjoy your life." What I want to say is, *Mara, don't leave me! You're my sister. We've been friends all these years.*

A farmer in coveralls limps by, dragging a small blond boy in a wagon. I throw my knapsack of beans, wheat berries, and cornmeal over my shoulder and follow Rachel. Each step away feels like something is ripping.

CHAPTER 11

Fool

The whole way down Route 119, past Speed, Gandeeville, and Snake
Hollow, I'm thinking about a baby that died at a homebirth in Hardy
County, on summer solstice, the longest day of the year.

*What am I doing in this new Ford station wagon being whipped back and
forth as we race through the night? What am I doing even going to deliveries
when our community is falling apart?*

The driver, a clean-shaven stranger, the minister of the Spencer
Seventh-Day Adventist Church, handles his late-model vehicle like a
racecar, and sitting in back, with the winding road and the new-car
smell, I'm about to puke.

Yesterday, Fern called and told me that word on the West Virginia
homebirth hotline is that the fetal death happened during labor. The
baby got stuck. When the head came out, the midwife tried everything,
squatting, hands and knees, pressure on the pubic bone. She even tried
to turn the baby with the screw maneuver that I've read about in *Wil-
liams Obstetrics*, but nothing worked.

You'd think I'd have more concern about the devastated family and
the poor birth attendant; that my heart would go out to them. Instead,
my eyes got steely and I asked Fern for the obstetrical details: "Were
there risks for shoulder dystocia?" "Any sign of gestational diabetes?"
"Had the mother ever delivered a large infant before?" What I'm really
asking is, "Were there any predictive factors? Is there a way to prevent
such a terrible outcome?"

All I could learn was that Jade, the primary birth attendant, called the
squad to take the mom to the hospital with the little baby's blue head
still sticking out, but it was too late. Of course it was too late . . .

This is the first bad outcome in the state's loosely knit network of
homebirth midwives and it will be investigated by the state coroner's

office for sure. Jade is sick with grief and fear. Homebirths, by midwives, are legal in West Virginia as long as we don't charge money, but birth at home isn't sanctioned, either, and there's no doubt there will be some kind of repercussions. We are all scared.

Now, here I am hurling down this snake of a road on my way to some stranger's house to do another home delivery. *What am I thinking? Am I prepared for this kind of responsibility? Do I imagine Jade has a monopoly on tragedy?*

We pass the sign to Bear Fork and, a few hairpin turns later, Wolf Run. Tom puts his arm around me. He knows how nauseated I get on a curvy road, and he knows about the baby's death. He also knows how fragile and forlorn I've felt since Mara's announcement that she and Benny are leaving the ridge. His hand on my shoulder says everything. He and I are solid. We are in this together. The commune may come and go but we are for always.

꙰

Another horseshoe twist and I urgently wind down the window and watch as my pinto bean supper covers the side of the pastor's shiny burgundy auto. "Sorry," I mumble, wiping my mouth with the back of my hand. The pastor, worried about getting me to the birth on time, doesn't even pull over. Ten minutes later, we screech into the drive of a pleasant brick ranch house. The front door flies open and light streams out on the porch.

"Oh, Patsy," Mr. Blundell, a pale, balding forty-year-old, erupts through the opening with a ragged sigh. "Praise Jesus, you got here! She's having a pretty hard time." I glance around the living room. Kids' colorful plastic toys are everywhere, but I don't hear any children's voices. They must be spending the night with grandparents.

Ordinarily I insist on a home visit before attending a birth, but because I injured my back, delivered two other babies, and started work for Community Action, there wasn't time. Now I see the results of my hastiness. I'm walking into the home of a family I barely know, have met only once. I have more enthusiasm than sense. *Fool. Fool.*

"Mr. Blundell, this is my husband, Tom." Blundell nods and shakes hands with Tom, glad to have another man around. The perspiring pastor beats a hasty retreat out the front door, saying he'll pray for us, and Jay Blundell immediately leads the way down the carpeted hall.

FAITH

At the door to the dark master bedroom, I see Bonnie crouched in an unmade bed. *This doesn't look good.* She reaches out, opening and closing her hand in a silent plea for me to come closer, then groans and grabs my fingers until the bones crunch. I notice a wet towel on the floor, soiled with brown amniotic fluid as thick and dark as beef gravy. "When did your water break?" I ask when the contraction lets up.

"Three days ago."

"Three days! Has it been that color all along?" The woman stares at the linen.

"I didn't notice . . . No. I don't think so. It was clear this morning. I called my OB in Charleston when I started leaking . . . that was Wednesday. He knows I was planning a homebirth and told me if I didn't have a fever, it was all right to stay home."

I am both impressed and appalled: impressed because it's rare in West Virginia to find a physician who's supportive of a woman giving birth at home; and appalled because after twenty-four hours with ruptured membranes the risk of infection goes up. It's been three days! Bonnie should have contacted me. I would have come to her. I might have recommended castor oil or intermittent nipple stimulation to get things moving. I would certainly have asked her what color her amniotic fluid was.

"Oh no, here's another one!" The woman grabs my hand again.

When she's done, I sit down on the bed. "Bonnie, I need to check you. The color of your water isn't normal. That brown is meconium, baby poop. It could mean danger for the infant. If there's time we need to get to the hospital."

"The hospital. No! Our baby is OK. God will protect . . ." She breaks off her sentence and rolls on her hands and knees. "My back! My back!" I press on her sacrum with the flat of my hand.

❦

"Hey, Bonnie, you look like you feel a lot better. Is it time?" It's nervous Jay Blundell, standing with Tom at the bedroom door, holding a pack of sterilized bedding in his outstretched arms. Bonnie shoots him a look, as if her pain is his fault. Tom takes in the chaotic scene and turns on the bedside light.

"We're going to find out right now how close she is," I tell the father as I pull on sterile gloves. "But I'm concerned about something." I catch Tom's eye, wanting him to know how serious this is but not wanting to freak out the family.

As the woman lies back and spreads her legs, I continue. "Bonnie's been leaking for three days, and at some time the amniotic fluid turned brown. This means the baby has pooped in its water. It's called meconium and is potentially dangerous. If the infant aspirates the poop as he's born, he can experience respiratory distress." I would like to add *and babies sometimes die of this,* but bite down on my lower lip when I find that Bonnie's cervix is already almost fully dilated, just a rim left.

"This is Bonnie's third baby," I explain to the couple. "She's going to deliver in the next thirty minutes. I thought we might try to get to the hospital, but there's no time."

That's probably why my hospital transfer rate is so low. My patients all progress too fast or call me too late. Then there are the bad country roads and the long distances to the hospitals to consider . . .

How did I get into this? You break one rule: always make a home visit. You break another few rules: take time to get to know the family and be sure they understand what you expect of them. It's a slippery slope, and you wind up risking an infant's life by delivering at home with thick meconium-stained fluid.

I worry my jaw back and forth while I check fetal heart tones. Tom, silent, understanding what's at stake, lays out the birth equipment. There's the usual olive oil, gauze, two sterilized hemostats, a blue suction bulb, a pair of scissors, and a cord clamp that looks like a girl's plastic hair barrette, and, lastly, though I've never even opened the package before, a sterile DeLee suction trap.

"The baby's heartbeat sounds great and he or she will be here in a few minutes, but when he comes out," I warn the couple, "I won't try to make him cry right away. I purposely won't stimulate him." I hold up the DeLee catheter. "With this plastic tube, we'll try to suck the meconium out of the baby's mouth before he has a chance to breathe. The filter will catch the brown mucus." I hand the clear plastic apparatus to Tom, who looks it over. He's a musical-instrument repairman, a carpenter, a mechanic, and a father; the suction trap doesn't faze him.

I can't tell how Bonnie and Jay are taking all this, or if they're even listening. Contractions are coming one after the other and Jay prays into his wife's ear. "The Lord is my shepherd, I shall not want . . ."

"Oh, heavenly Jesus, I got to push!" That's Bonnie.

"Warm compresses." Tom holds out the bowl.

"He maketh me to lie down in green pastures . . ." That's Jay.

"It's coming! Oh God, it's coming!" Bonnie again.

Furious activity.

"Lay down now, Bonnie! Here on your side. Jay, hold her leg. Blow! Blow! Ready with the DeLee?" The head's hanging out of the vagina. Everything stops. Dead silence.

Tom calmly leans over and suctions the baby's mouth with the vinyl tube, as if he's done this before. I flash for a second on what it must have been like for Jade, the midwife, when her patient's baby got stuck, then I take the fragile skull between my two hands and gently push down. *First shoulder out.* Up now. *Second shoulder out.* Carefully, I lay the chalky newborn on the sheets. It looks dead, but it's only *not here yet* and we want it that way. As promised, we make no effort to stimulate until my husband suctions again and then looks up with a wide smile.

"No meconium in the mouth or throat."

"All right, little one. Time to breathe!" Dawn is just creeping under the curtains. I blow on the infant's belly. The breath of life I call it. The baby gasps when the cool air hits her abdomen and she lets out a wail.

"My baby. My Faith!" That's Bonnie.

"Praise Jesus!" That's Jay.

The tiny girl opens her eyes.

Reckoning

The smell of new-cut hay through the Volvo's open windows reminds me that summer is more than half over as I wind along Johnson Creek after my fourth visit with Etta Utt.

White clapboard homes with pots of red geraniums and neatly mowed yards line the side of the blacktop road, but I am not really seeing them. My churning mind turns to Mara.

On the farm, we go on with our work. We tend the garden, mulch our young apple orchard, and cut winter wood, but never talk about our friends' decision to move into Spencer. What's there to say? Benny and Mara are leaving. Once community surrounded me like a warm quilt. Now the quilt is mostly holes.

When I turn off the pavement onto Snake Run, everything changes. The gravel road is rough and rutted. I've just landed in the third world. Worn mobile homes on cement blocks sit in overgrazed fields. In every yard there's a pig or two, an outhouse, a tilting barn, and the inevitable body of a broken-down vehicle being saved for parts. I stare hard at the ramshackle dwellings, not believing people live there.

I, who have chosen voluntary poverty . . . I, who have elected to live without running water, plumbing, or electricity, I, who only recently had a phone installed, am shocked to see families existing without the basic conveniences of the twentieth century. These are homes right out of the Great Depression.

I recall the Walker Evans photographs taken for the Farm Security Administration in the 1930s, the gaunt, sad-faced women standing on falling-down porches. Nothing has changed. That's what I'm thinking when, in a tight curve just past the cemetery, a mammoth water truck rumbles around the bend in the narrow road.

There are ditches and trees on either side, nowhere to pull over . . . I slam my eyes shut, stomp on the brake, flash on Mica and Orion's faces, and brace for the inevitable. There's the crash of metal. Glass flies everywhere. The front end of the Volvo crumples like a wad of paper but the safety belt holds as my neck jerks forward and back.

After that, silence . . .

❧

It's the insistent *chirp-chirp* of a tiny wren that alerts me I'm not dead. With my eyes squeezed shut, I find myself still sitting in the Volvo's comfortable upholstered seat with my hands braced on the steering wheel. I check my limbs, clinch my fists, and wiggle my toes. *I have feeling . . . without searing pain. That seems good.* Then I notice the sound of the motor still running and blink my eyes open. The air reeks of gasoline, and through the shattered windshield I see black smoke.

Fumbling frantically with the safety restraint, I manage to crawl out, stagger into a ditch, and collapse on the grass.

❧

"You OK, honey?" A white-haired woman with gray rhinestone bifocals bends over me. She wears a black dress, old black grandma shoes, and dark hose. The rail-thin driver of the water truck hobbles toward us. It's hard to tell if he's been injured, or has walked like this for years.

"You OK, honey?" the lady asks again and places one wrinkled hand on my arm.

"Yeah, I'm fine." *I am not really fine and our blue Volvo, uninsured, is totaled.*

"Shit, I'm sorry," the other driver curses. "There was no way I could get over or brake in time."

"My old man is calling the sheriff. Do we need an ambulance too?" the lady interrupts.

"No, I'm going to be all right . . . really. My shoulder hurts but nothing's bleeding, nothing's broke. How about you?" I turn back to the middle-aged fellow who wears jeans, a two-day-old beard, and a Southern States Farm Co-op cap low over his eyes.

He shrugs and pushes his hat back, but skips my question. "God, I'm sorry as hell. These roads is too narrow. You're sure you're all right?" He kneels next to me.

I try to stand up to show them I'm fine, but my legs buckle, so I sit back down. "Could someone call my husband? He's home with the kids."

"Hobart!" the lady shouts to her mate, who's watching the scene from the sloping porch of the faded green trailer across the road. "Get over here with a pencil and paper. This girl wants you to call someone."

Thirty minutes later, I'm sitting in Mr. and Mrs. Wheeler's trailer on their brown plaid sofa with a flowered plate of cookies on my lap and a cup of strong tea in a mug at my side. The living room smells like Lysol and there isn't a dust bunny anywhere. From outside the worn mobile home, I hadn't imagined such a tranquil interior.

The silenced TV across the room shows pictures of the first test-tube baby, Louise Brown. I'm transfixed. She looks entirely normal, a cute kid. Then I catch sight of myself in a silver framed mirror over the television and am startled to see a woman I hardly recognize, pale, with disheveled short hair sticking up at all angles. I smooth it down.

"So you're the midwife," Mrs. Wheeler confirms. "We'd heard about you at the Seventh Day Adventist Church." I'm just about to ask what they heard, bad or good, when Tom appears at the screen door.

"It wasn't the little lady's fault," Hobart Wheeler says in my defense when my husband sits down. "I was here on the porch. Saw the whole thing. Been an accident on that turn every year as long as I can remember. We told the state highway department least three times, but they don't listen. County highway superintendent says they'll come by and check. I wouldn't hold my breath. They won't come 'til someone gets killed." Tom and I catch each other's eyes again. We don't need words to understand . . . *that someone could have been me.*

An hour later, we sit in the jeep in the dark at the end of Steel Hollow. The full moon is just rising over the hills. *Whip-poor-will. Whip-poor-will,* a night bird sings. When I finally begin to cry, I'm not sure if I weep because our first good car, the Volvo, is totaled, because Mara and Benny are leaving the commune, or because the world is so beautiful and I'm not dead.

"I'm so sorry about the car," I tell Tom. "I'm so sorry." Before us the valley is a huge bowl of light. He holds me in his arms and I cry, deep gulping sobs; then he presses our foreheads together.

CHAPTER 12

Falling Star

"Did you see that? A falling star! It went clear across the sky to Steele Hollow." Tom and I lie alone in the middle of the horseshoe ridge, under a moonless sky, with a silk banner of tiny lights above us. Orion and Mica are already in bed and Rachel is babysitting. I shake my head no, meaning I missed the meteor, and stare off where Tom points.

Seen a shooting star tonight . . . He sings a few bars of an old Dylan song, then turns on his side and pushes my bangs back from my eyes. "I know you're sad about the community. There's not much left."

Rachel's little clapboard house was finished right on schedule, August 20. Though the twelve-by-twelve two-story dwelling is not yet insulated, the windows are tight and she has a door, a blue one we trash-picked from the Roane County dump.

In her ritual move to her new place, we followed Snow White like the Seven Dwarfs, marching up through the woods, carrying books and bedding, boxes of papers, and the used dishes she scored at a Methodist Church yard sale. As we trooped inside her new house, I flicked my gaze up to her roof, where Tom almost lost his life falling two stories onto the lumber pile, and thanked the Great Spirit for saving him.

Rachel asked us to bless the cabin, so while Laurel read a passage from *The Prophet,* I surveyed her abode. Tom built the table and Rachel made her own benches. There's a wooden counter but no sink yet, just two tin washbowls. There are bookshelves near the door and a ladder that leads to the loft. Her bed is upstairs. She'll be cozy enough, but I'll miss her gingerbread and maybe even her nighttime fiddle playing . . .

A few days later, Mara and Benny moved to *their* new home, at dusk, without any ceremony. It was raining and thunder threatened in the west. We loaded their worldly goods in the back of the Jeep pickup and Tom drove them to town. There was no joking around, no cries of good luck. All this happened after I quit my job for lack of a reliable vehicle and just before Laurel announced, as we harvested the potatoes in the garden, that she was thinking of joining a folk dance troupe in Philadelphia this winter.

♈

I'm on my knees with my hands in the dirt and look up, shocked. I had no idea Laurel too was thinking of leaving.

"I'm tired of grubbing in the earth," she tries to explain. "Of always being cold or hot or dirty." I start to cry, and when I wipe my tears I get mud on my face. *Laurel is leaving!* I'm not just crying for myself, but for Stacy and Mica . . . for all of us.

♈

I shift on the grass, still staring up at the stars, next to Tom. A bobcat screeches twice down in the hollow, a sound like a woman crying. Tom takes my hand. "I'm sad about the community, too, but doesn't it seem cozy to have our own place? I think we might be happier this way. I like it."

Why does this guy always have to be so optimistic? His cup's always full. Mine leaks like a sieve.

"I tried that nuclear-family scene once before, in Minnesota, remember?"

"But the falling star is a *sign,* Pats." Tom flops back with a chuckle and extends his arms.

I know he doesn't believe in signs and I don't see anything positive about the dissolution of our commune. It's a slow landslide and there's no way to stop the erosion. We'll just finish the trim on Rachel's little cottage, get it insulated, then preserve our food for the winter . . . then . . . I don't know . . . For the first time in years, I'm out of visions, out of dreams.

"Did I tell you the Marathon Natural Gas guy that takes care of the well at the corner of Anne Margaret's land, Mr. Vogler, asked me if I wanted to be on the Roane County Emergency Squad?"

"You didn't say anything." I take a deep breath and attempt to blow away my bad vibes.

"It's a volunteer squad, with only a few paid workers, but the EMT course is free. I thought it would be something I could do, meet some local people, and maybe eventually even earn some money. Classes are held at the hospital. I'd have to go in every night for two weeks. Mr. Vogler said he'd pick me up."

I shrug. "Sounds all right, especially if it doesn't cost anything." Tom spoons around me in the dry grass, but I'm stiff as a board. Above us, a million stars, tiny silver nails, wound the night.

Work Party

The sun is just rising over the hills. *Morning has broken, like the first morning,* we sing as we bounce up Trippet Run in the back of the jeep. Goldenrod and deep purple aster line the road. It's almost like the old photo, pinned to the wall in the kitchen, the one of the truck filled with happy communards, laughing, full of visions of the new world.

"Hold on tight," I tell Mica. I know it isn't safe to ride in the pickup bed, but since the Volvo accident, the jeep truck is all we have.

I turn to look in the cab window where Mara sits holding baby Orion with Ben on one side and Stacy on the other. Her hair's almost as long as mine before I chopped off my braids. I can't hear what they're saying, but Stacy, who's driving, laughs and thumps the steering wheel. Tom isn't with us. He's working a twenty-four-hour shift with the emergency squad as part of his EMT training. *Black birds have spoken, like the first birds* . . . Rachel, Laurel, Mica, and I sing in the back.

At the end of Tripplet, where the dirt road dead-ends under the pines, we park and walk along the top of the hill for a quarter of a mile. You can smell the downfalls before you see them, sweet, warm, and alcoholic.

First we collect the fruit still hanging, golden globules of light. There aren't many without wormholes or scabs, but the best are gently placed in baskets to carry back to the truck and will be stored in the root cellar on beds of straw. The rest we dump in buckets to make dried apples, applesauce, and apple cider. I wipe one on the back of my pants and take a big bite. Crunchy, sweet and sour! *Thank you, apple tree!*

All morning we fill our crates and baskets, making trips back and forth to the jeep. It's a treasure hunt, like trash-picking, only better, because no storeowner or cop is going to chase us away. Orion fusses and I let him out of the baby carrier to crawl in the yellow grass while we have lunch.

"Think that's wise?" Laurel asks.

I look around. What does she mean? Is she concerned about the rocky soil? Is she worried about reptiles? Just this summer, a copperhead bit our hippie neighbor, Tobbie, who lives on the other side of Steele Hollow. She was walking barefoot at dusk, going out to the pasture to check on her horse. She got an anti-venom shot at Roane General. Without it she would have lost her foot, or maybe her life.

"The yellow jackets . . ." Laurel glances with dramatic eyes at the feisty stinging insects that swarm over the fallen fruit. She's right. A yellow jacket's sting is worse than a bee's. I pick Orion up, wondering what to do with him.

"Here." Mara reaches out. Our one-year-old leaps into her arms. "My back is tired. I'll go up to the truck and change his diapers."

This is what I love about raising children in community. It's not just up to me. Everyone looks out for our little boys. It's one of the things I will miss most. I wonder how women who live in nuclear families survive . . . I guess I'll find out . . .

I watch Mara waddle up the trail. Sometimes I forget how pregnant she is. Eight months is a little far along for this work. As her midwife, shouldn't I be taking better care of her? On the other hand, pioneer women did much harder labor.

Ben and Stacy, imitating angry gorillas, climb the tree above us as high as they can and shake the brittle old branches. Rachel and I laugh as the fruit falls on our heads. Mica's snatching up apples as if we're on an Easter egg hunt. When all the usable fruit has been gathered and packed in a bucket or basket, we leave the rest for the deer and head back.

Tom has missed this good day, but I trust he's enjoying his emergency medical training. I climb into the pickup bed with our harvest, zip up my jacket against the cool evening, and pull Mica into my lap. Orion is again riding up front with Mara.

The pickup rumbles and bumps over the ruts as the sun drops into waves of red. No one tries to talk over the engine noise. Feeling like Midas, I survey our precious treasure of gold; but who will be left on the farm to eat it?

Fall Returns

CHAPTER 13

Siren

I sweep the honey-colored pine floor, wipe off the table, then slide into Rachel's old room, now the new bathroom in the Long House.

"Isn't it pretty?" I ask Orion, who's riding in the back carrier while I work. Our enamel potty sits in the corner on a remnant of gold and green linoleum, trash-picked from behind McIntosh Hardware. Yellow flowered curtains hang in the window. There's a clothesline for laundry, my old green woven rag rug that Ila made me on her loom, and, best of all, an actual porcelain bathtub that Tom discovered in the Shoepecks' dump. All we are missing is indoor plumbing.

We still have to carry and heat bathwater, but it drains through a pipe in the floor, and what a luxury, to recline in warm liquid instead of standing up in a galvanized washtub! Mica and Orion can even play in their bath, a treat they've never had.

🜚

"Why'd you let me sleep so long?" Tom complains as he comes down the ladder. "I wanted to finish the insulation on the back of Rachel's house."

The Roane County Emergency Squad has hired Tom on a regular basis. He's now taking two twenty-four-hour shifts each week and sleeps until noon the next day. Together we studied the thick Emergency Management workbook from front to back. I'd never seen him so focused. The laid-back hippie Tom was suddenly inhabited by a new guy, sharp, disciplined, confident.

"I was down there this morning with Stacy and Laurel," I explain. "It's almost done. You can finish what's left after lunch . . . How'd it go last night? I heard the siren in the distance about midnight."

Orion reaches for his daddy and Tom takes him, balancing him on his head with one hand and clip-clopping around the room like a horse. Orion squeals with delight and Tom's grumpy mood evaporates.

"Everything go OK?" I've become intensely interested in my companion's new medical life and quiz him for every detail.

"Not really. You know old Mr. Nutter . . . goes to Steele Hollow Church with Sadie Shoepeck and her family? He used to be the pastor there." I shake my head no. Tom sits down on the bench, now serious. "Yeah you do, we met him when we went to the chapel to sing. He lives way out on Tripplet. I was partnered with Mr. Vogler last night. We came up Steele Hollow and then took the dirt road almost out to the orchard. The old man was dead when we got there. Massive heart attack. Maybe a stroke. I knew when I saw him that it was too late.

"But that wasn't the worst," my husband goes on.

"Not the worst? How can it get any worse than picking up a dead guy?"

"Well, we transported Mr. Nutter to the Sinett Funeral Home by 2:30 a.m. and were just back in bed when we got a second call, a fight down at the Road House, that place along Route 33, the joint with the strippers. The state cops were there. Some babe thought her husband was cheating and came down with his rifle and shot him in the arm. While we were trying to get the bleeding stopped, the woman was still trying to attack him. The scene was out of control. They say these kind of domestic situations happen all the time."

I glance at the window seat where Tom threw his shirt when he got home; the new blue long-sleeved uniform shirt with the patch I'd proudly sewn on the sleeve. For the first time, I notice the dried blood on the front.

"Do you still want to do this?" I stare at my friend, the father of our child, stroking his baby's fuzzy head. He looks tired, big circles under his eyes, with a two-day-old beard. He had to shave when he joined the squad. Tom stands and tosses Orion into the air. The baby throws out his arms, laughing.

"Sure, it was great!" He follows my gaze to the bloody garment and flashes a grin. "But we'll have to get a few more EMS shirts."

DYLAN

"Finally!" I squeal.

"Shhhhh." That's Tom. He doesn't want me to wake Orion. It's 6:00 a.m. and I'm on the phone with Mara, who's two weeks past due.

"Is the fluid clear?" I've become paranoid about meconium since the Blundell birth, and meconium-stained fluid is more common in overdue pregnancies.

"I think so, but it just keeps trickling. I put on a pad," Mara tells me.

"Contractions?"

"I'm not sure. They don't hurt, but my abdomen gets tight clear up to my neck. I've been up and down to the bathroom all night. Nice to have a flush toilet instead of an outhouse."

ϔ

A few hours later, I'm checking Mara on her bed upstairs in their new house on the state mental hospital grounds. A worn green and white patchwork quilt covers the hand-me-down full-size double-spring bed, a housewarming present from Sadie Shoepeck. Benny has set up some board and brick bookshelves, and in the corner stands a white crib they bought at a yard sale.

"So, tonight sometime?" Ben asks, sitting on the corner of the mattress, holding Mara's hand. I notice that he's cut his curly hair short and now trims his beard. "Sorry if we made you come too early."

"It's OK. Things might go quicker than you think."

They don't go quicker. All day Mara walks the bare hardwood floors, squats and slow dances with her husband, but mostly stands leaning over the bathroom sink swaying her hips and looking into Benny's brown eyes in the medicine-chest mirror. Her face is pink and her golden hair is coming out of her ponytail. She looks beautiful and strong, the way women look in labor when they aren't afraid.

Ben rubs her lower back. Laurel sits on the toilet seat and massages Mara's legs to keep her loose. I stand at the bathroom door, watching, thinking it's too bad you have to have a baby to get all this attention. Then, about dawn, without warning, Mara hits the floor on her hands and knees, moaning and wagging her bottom like a dog. "God, that was a hard one. I want to push!" I notice blood trickling down one leg.

"Better lie down so I can check you. It may be time."

"No shit?" says Ben, running his fingers through his short hair so it stands on end. "You really think so?" Tom and Stacy watch from the doorway. Rachel, with Orion on her hip, slips by, her dark eyes asking if everything's OK.

✻

An hour later the warm room is crowded with cheerleaders, Tom, Stacy, Rachel and the boys . . . Laurel wipes Mara's red face after each contraction. Tom pours warm olive oil over my fingers as I massage her perineum.

"I've figured it out," Mara tells us. "If I growl at the beginning, even if I don't have the urge to push, once the baby starts moving, the urge follows and my uterus takes over and makes me bear down."

"Grrrrrr!" she demonstrates.

"Grrrrrr!" Rachel growls, too, finally finding her role.

Thirty minutes later. "Oh, it *stings*. Oh, Patsy, it burns bad!"

"Pant, Mara! Pant!" Everyone in the room pants with her, their eyes riveted on the emerging new life.

Mara delivers the infant into my hands, first the head with its chubby cheeks, then the shoulders, then the rest. Her body works perfectly to produce this new life and I remember that this is the way it's supposed to be. This is the way, if not interfered with, most women can give birth.

Laurel pulls open the blinds, and everyone blinks as the golden sun pours into the room. *Like the first morning,* I think. Mica crawls on the bed to say hello. Orion watches from the child carrier on Tom's back. Mara reaches out for her baby. "It's Dylan, right?" She looks up at Benny and laughs.

CHAPTER 14

Rebirth

"I hope my shirt's dry." Tom clomps up the ladder, shakes the wrinkles out of his uniform, and stands buttoning it in the bedroom doorway. I'm folding laundry with Orion on the bed. I observe that after three washings, the bloodstains on his EMS shirt are gone.

"You like your job?" I know he does. I just like to hear about it.

He drops down beside me to help match the socks, our big wool ones, Mica's little-boy tube socks, and Orion's tiny cotton ones. "The runs are scary sometimes and hanging around the station gets boring, but I told you about the fight at the rooming house didn't I? Two old guys in Spencer beat each other almost senseless. One man's face was kicked in so bad you could hardly recognize him as human.

"It's hard when we don't have a paramedic with us . . . someone to start an IV. Like that run with the gunshot at the Road House; the guy might have died if Vogler hadn't been there. He and Molliann are the only paramedics in town and they each only work two twenty-four-hour shifts, so three days a week, the emergency medical technicians are on their own. I've watched them both put in the intravenous catheter and think I could do it, but an EMT isn't certified for IVs."

Tom's confidence about such technical procedures amazes me. Though I knew he was good at fixing things—old trucks, musical instruments, windup alarm clocks, and kerosene lanterns—I wouldn't have dreamed he had an aptitude for fixing *people,* or the ability to learn so quickly.

The Tom I've always known is this loose hippie bass player, a quiet long-haired dude in the background, someone you can rely on without ever realizing how intelligent, fearless, and competent he is.

"What would you do if you were *without* Vogler and thought a patient might bleed to death? Would you have the guts to just start an IV? I mean, without being a trained paramedic?"

Tom looks up from tying his boots. He's shaved his beard, just left a mustache so you can actually see the cleft in his chin, and I understand now why women are attracted to men in uniform.

"Probably try to get the needle in. It's important to get a line started before the victim loses too much blood and his veins collapse. I might get fired for it though."

"Maybe not, if you saved someone's life. They might give you a commendation!" He knows I'm kidding. The way most bureaucracies work, he'd most likely get canned.

He changes the subject. "I heard Molliann tell someone that Community Action has funding for grants to the LPN program at Arch Moore Vocational School."

"LPN, like a licensed practical nurse? Maybe Rachel would be interested."

"No, I mean *you*. Community Action would pay a salary while you went to school. We could use the money. I'm sure you'd get in."

I snort a short laugh, flashing on a vision of me as Florence Nightingale. "I can just see me with a little nurse's cap and white stockings!"

Tom pulls on his new blue zip-up EMT jacket. He bends to kiss the baby, who's curled on his side in our big bed, almost asleep. "Well, think about it." He gently kisses Orion without waking him. "I'll stop and say good-bye to Mica up at the Little House."

When he leaves, I put away the laundry, carefully stacking the clothes and diapers on our new wooden shelves. Then I stroll around the kids' room picking up toys. I stop when I notice my green journal and pull out an envelope. I'm surprised that Tom and I are thinking along the same lines. Actually I'm dreaming a few steps ahead.

Since meeting Etta Utt and the other mothers on my rounds for Community Action, I've begun to feel strongly that I want to take care of a wider variety of women, not just the healthy, low-risk, homesteading hippie women I've been privileged to serve. There are so many others that deserve tender, respectful care. I've already sent for, and received back in the mail, a pamphlet on how to become a certified nurse-midwife.

Sue Ellen's breech delivery, the Blundell birth with meconium, and the death of the baby at the homebirth in Harper County have also affected me. I need more training. I sit on the edge of the bed and read through the flyer again.

To be a nurse-midwife, I'd need to go back to school, become an RN, and then most likely get my master's degree. The program would take three or four years and we would have to leave the farm and West Virginia . . . *I have two kids and no money . . . It doesn't seem likely.*

From a distance I hear a siren and picture Tom behind the wheel of the Roane County ambulance. He flicks on the flashing light and speeds out Route 33. The siren gets closer, then fades away.

Beelzebub

Winter is coming and Tom and Mica are working down in the woods, cutting dead pine for firewood. "Timber!" yells Tom. *"Timmberrrrr!"* echoes Mica, dragging it out like a lumberjack.

Not wanting to go out in the cold to the privy, I squat over the white porcelain potty in our new bathroom. If I'd used the outhouse, I might not have seen the six-inch-long parasite that emerged from my body. It lays on top of my stool.

"Tom!" I scream, peeking though my fingers.

There are moments in your life when, like a movie, things go into slow motion. The worm wiggles sensually . . . *I'm a straight-A honor student who went to Girls State for God's sake! I'm a midwife who eats all organic food. This can't be happening!*

"Tom!!" I scream louder and look through my fingers. *It's still there.*

Over the years on the commune, we've experienced such third world afflictions as pinworms, impetigo, chiggers, head lice, and scabies; but a large roundworm is the last straw. Hearing my calls, Tom and Mica run in and stare down. Mica covers a little grin but my husband knows better than to laugh at me. I'm bawling my head off. *"This is it!"* I yell and pull up my jeans. "I can't take it anymore. I can't do this."

"Settle down, Pats." Tom lays his hand on me. "We'll get medicine in town."

"Call now," I demand. "We want the *strongest* prescription."

"I'll phone Dr. Dan in the morning. His office is already closed. I'm gonna make dinner now." Mica's still patting my arm, and Orion, hearing his mother scream, has big eyes.

"Don't make any food for me. I'd just be feeding the worms!"

I collapse on the window seat in the main room and put the baby to breast, more for my comfort than his, then pull Mica down beside me. "This is miserable, bud."

"I know a song!" Mica's blue eyes light up as he tries to cheer me. "I learned it from kids at the co-op."

"Mmmm." I'm too busy feeling sorry for myself to be interested.

Nobody loves me, everybody hates me, Mica chants in a singsong voice. I remember that song. I sang it when I was a kid, too. *I think I'll go eat worms.*

"Nooooo!" I roll over and tickle Mica to get him to stop. Sometimes you have to laugh or you'll cry. I'm laughing *and* crying. Orion smiles and drools milk, sensing a joke.

Big ones, little ones, Mica goes on. *Fat ones, skinny ones . . .*

Cleansed

For a week I can't eat. We buy enough Mebendazole for everyone in the commune, just in case I'm not the only one riddled with parasites. Ronna, another of Colin's friends from Chicago, who showed up three days ago to check out the commune, gets a pass on the meds. The thin forty-year-old, a former literature professor looking for a new life, hasn't been here long enough to be considered potentially wormy. Rachel has generously offered the woman a place in her loft.

I take an extra dose of the Mebendazole, sixteen tablets in all. Tom reads from our worn copy of *Where There Is No Doctor* that 25 percent of the world population is infected with roundworms, but it doesn't make me feel better. Some might say my response to the organism is exaggerated, that it's no big deal. That's because they've never seen a six-inch . . . live . . . wriggling . . . roundworm come out of *their* body.

After each trip to the outhouse, I check to see if another parasite emerges, but I never find one and neither does anyone else. The dreadfulness fades, but not much.

Then rains come. With Mara's birth and the worm crisis, I hadn't even noticed the change in the season. Oddly, I now feel spiritually cleansed, as if I've hit bottom. I've forgotten my dream of going to nurse-midwifery school. There are no homebirths coming up for at least two months. We're just living each day and then going to bed.

CHAPTER 15

Flying

With care, I fold our best clothes and stuff them into a knapsack. I'm packing for a four-day excursion, a mini-vacation in Athens, Ohio, that Tom arranged, because he knows how low I've been since Mara left and the parasite made its appearance.

The plan seems to be having the desired effect. *Some glad day when this life is over, I'll fly away,* I sing as I pack.

We haven't been on a trip like this since our honeymoon, when we hitchhiked to Williamsburg, snuck into the grounds of Colonial National Historical Park, and slept illegally in a tent under a bridge. Mara and Ben have offered to take the boys, as a gift for my delivering Dylan.

Tom comes up behind me and tosses me on the bed. "Hey, cut it out!" We're both feeling giddy, rolling around, messing up the quilt. "I can take you easy, buster." I'm sitting on his stomach, pretending I've pinned him.

"You're all mouth and no action." Tom rolls me off with ease, holds me down, and gives me a long kiss. "Come on, you've packed enough. Let's hit the road. The Knotts will be gone for a week and they have a washer and dryer." The Knotts are the Quaker family he stayed with when he used to fix instruments in Athens at the music store.

❧

"Good morning, flying squirrel," I call out as a small soaring rodent sails across our path and lands spread out on the trunk of a maple before us. It's a chilly day with a clear sky, no leaves on the trees, but the grass on the ridge is green from the rains. A few goldenrods still droop on their stems. My good mood bubbles over.

Some glad morning when this life is over, I'll fly away, I sing at top volume, as we tromp across the ridge and then along the partially finished road along Anne Margaret's fence line. An echo comes up from the hollow. *I'll fly away.*

"No smoke from the chimney," Tom observes, indicating her small cottage on the side of the hill. "Stacy told me Anne Margaret and Joshua went back to Chicago to see her parents and might stay awhile."

Two more people gone, I think. Ordinarily this would spin me into depression, but today I'm detached. *Just a few more weary days and then, I'll fly away* . . . The tune won't leave my head. As we reach our new old 1965 red Volvo that Tom bought for $300 with his EMT money, my lover joins the chorus and I do a little jig before I get in.

❦

Crossing Noble's Ridge, on Route 33, I study the Arch Moore Vocational Center, with its long, low brick buildings, the place where Tom suggested I attend the LPN course and get paid to go to school by the federal CETA program.

At first I resisted, unable to picture myself as a nurse, carrying a doctor's charts around, giving shots, and fluffing pillows, but two women friends from the food co-op have already signed up, and I finally sent for the application. It may be a path toward becoming a certified nurse-midwife. Not only that: we could sure use the money.

❦

Two hours later, as we cross the metal bridge over the Ohio River in Parkersburg, Tom breaks the quiet. "What do you want to do in Athens tonight?" I blink myself awake and squint at the traffic lights.

"Everything! Let's get dinner and then go to a movie. It must be five years since we've been to a flick."

"We took Mica to *Star Wars* in Spencer a year ago, remember?"

"Well, it was five years before that, then. And tomorrow you can take me to the music store where you used to work and I'll get some new guitar strings. Sunday I want to go to Quaker meeting."

❦

In Athens, we do all the things I hoped for, and more: shop for kids' clothes at the Salvation Army, trash-pick an old maple table we find on the sidewalk, watch mallards land in the blue-green water of Dow Lake. On Sunday, our last day in civilization, we wander over to the Ohio University library.

In a private glassed-in reading room, I rest my elbows on the scarred oak table. "So, what does Thomas Harman want to do with the rest of his life?" I tease, as if I'm a host on National Public Radio. I'm surprised when my husband answers seriously.

"I've been thinking . . . Remember when we were at the food co-op the other day, that couple from New York City that was talking about their ten-year plan? Nothing like that ever entered my mind. We've been so focused on *being here now,* but I like the idea. I've been asking myself, what would *I* like to do in the next ten years? I thought maybe I'd start by getting certified as a paramedic and eventually go to school to become a physician's assistant."

I'm taken aback by this revelation and a little pissed. "How come you didn't say anything?" *Like he's had a big discussion with himself and I've been left out . . .*

"I didn't want to get in a fight. I know how important the commune is to you."

"Since Laurel left for the dance troupe in Philadelphia there's not much commune left, just Rachel and Stacy and the kids, you and I and that new friend of Colin's, Ronna . . . if she decides to stay." I rest my chin on my hand. "Where would you go to school, anyway? Is there a program near Spencer?"

"Nah, that's the problem. Vogler says the closest paramedic classes are in Charleston or at Hocking College, a few miles north of Athens. This is just something I've been thinking about . . . I need employment we can count on. Carpentry isn't reliable and an EMT position is minimum wage."

I study my husband, seeing him in a new way, a man taking charge of his future. "Aren't you afraid of being co-opted by the system? Losing your ideals?"

He laughs through his nose. "No."

Above us, dust motes dance in the light through the tall, many-paned windows. I hadn't wanted to talk about my fantasy of becoming a nurse-midwife. It makes me feel disloyal to what's left of the community, as if we're plotting a getaway . . . but since he shared his dream . . .

"Well, I looked into the LPN program."

Tom tilts back in his chair and waits.

"If you get your LPN license at Arch Moore, you can get your RN in one more year at Parkersburg Community College." Now that I've started, my fantasies flow like water from a spring in the hillside.

"You need to be a registered nurse to become a certified nurse-midwife. We could do it, the two of us. I could open a birthing center. You could become a physician's assistant. We could start a free clinic."

Once I begin, I dream big, and Tom sits straight up in his chair. I almost skip to the reference desk, borrow a pencil and paper, and begin to sketch a collective future that we'd never imagined. *Can I really give myself permission after fifteen years of living in the most spartan manner, at Tolstoy Farm, CNVA, Chester Creek House, the Homestead in Minnesota, and on the ridge at No Name Farm, to make such a radical change? Is it possible?*

"We could move into Spencer this winter and rent a little house. I could apply to the LPN program and, if I get in, be paid by CETA. You could take care of the kids during the day while I go to school."

Tom breaks in, scratching the cleft in his chin. "In the spring we can move back to the farm, work the gardens and live in the Long House. I could continue as an EMT, a few nights a week, and when you're a nurse, you could support us while *I* go to school."

There are moments in your life when time speeds up like a film on fast-forward. This is one. We excitedly draw timelines and maps with circles of the distance we'll have to move from Roane County, the center of our world, if I'm to become a nurse-midwife and Tom's to become a paramedic or physician's assistant.

We have no idea how we'll pay for our education or how we'll take care of our children, but we are euphoric; we've done difficult things before. What's this compared to building log houses, cultivating fields with only hoes and spades, hauling water for a quarter of a mile, walking through blizzards? Nothing seems impossible.

�֍

Back on State Street, an outline of our ten-year plan folded in quarters and tucked in Tom's jeans, we sit on the edge of the fountain at the archway to the Ohio University campus. The smell of lamb and vegetables from the falafel cart on the corner reaches across the lawn. It's a warm night for November.

"If you didn't know us," I whisper to Tom, "you might think we were just hip university students, just playing flower children. You couldn't tell, by looking, what we've been through, the joy and the hardships."

This notion pleases me. "No one would know that just a few days ago, we were living like Guatemalan peasants or that a few weeks ago I expelled a *foot-long roundworm*." I'm exaggerating for effect and Tom smiles. It's the first time I've been able to make a joke about the parasite.

The streetlamps come on and shine down on the undergrads crossing the intersection near the student bookstore. "Come over here," I whisper, and lead Tom around the backside of the fountain. On a pile of leaves, we lie down in the shadows under a bare maple and look up at the sky. There's no sound but the cascading water, the cars moving down State Street, and a girl's distant laugh.

On our backs, we gaze up at the almost full moon. High overhead, there's the high-pitched barking of late geese heading south. I strain to see them, peering through a web of branches, and am suddenly falling into the sky, then sailing high across the green campus and over the silver river below. Like the flying squirrel, I soar, wheel across the rolling hills of southern Ohio, then over the steeper hills of West Virginia.

I see headlights below of semitrucks on the four-lane, then smaller lights of pickups on Route 33. Below, in Spencer, on the state hospital grounds, Mara and Benny are putting Mica and Orion and Dylan to bed in their two-story cottage.

I follow Steele Hollow Road up the ridge, my arms like wings, and circle low over the farm. Only one kerosene light shines golden out the window of the Little House, a tiny beacon of hope, where Stacy sits cross-legged on the floor playing the Autoharp for Rachel and the new woman, Ronna. *For the beauty of the earth* . . . they sing the old hymn.

For the glory of the skies. For the love which from our birth over and around us lies . . .

The bells in the tower of the Presbyterian church on Court Street are ringing the same song this evening. Tom and I know the words and sing the hymn together. *For the beauty of each hour, of the day and of the night.* He reaches for my hand and our palms fit together. *Spirit of all to thee we raise, this our song of grateful praise . . .*

FROM THE SILVER JOURNAL

❧

Cedar House on Hope Lake
2008–2009

❧

Spring

CHAPTER I

Night Call

"How bad?" Tom asks, rubbing his fingers through his short silver buzz.

Not a good first line, and I shut my eyes tight. I wasn't always this way, afraid of night phone calls. It was the years of teenage rebellion that did it. There were calls from the cops, calls from other parents, calls from the ER. If my boys didn't end up in prison they would end up dead, that's what I feared . . .

I sit straight up in our king-sized pillow-topped bed and turn on the light.

"Is there much blood?" *Definitely not a good second line.* "OK, admit her short stay. I'll see her in the morning. But don't give her any more narcotics. Her surgery was over three weeks ago." He hands the phone back and I place it into the charger.

"What?"

"It's a chronic-pelvic-pain patient that I did a laparoscopy on almost a month ago. She's having vaginal bleeding. Probably just a period, but she's carrying on so much, the ER doc doesn't want to send her home." Tom turns off the light and adjusts his pillow. Already his breathing slows, but I'm still wide awake, pulsing with adrenaline. It's 2:45 a.m.

I stare around our bedroom, a space so large it could hold the whole Minnesota log cabin.

Outside, faint moonlight shines through the trees, pours into the room through the floor-to-ceiling windows, lays shadows across the floor. Pulling on my long white terry bathrobe, I pad across the carpet. A ghost woman nods from the reflection in the glass. In the likeness, you can't see the gray streaks in my short, once chestnut, hair, or the faint worry lines over my nose. You can't see my blue eyes, still round when I get excited, or the pink cheeks, but it's still me, the girl with long braids.

As I pass our dresser, I feel for my prayer box, a small, round, red wooden container with stars and the moon on the lid. My three boys' names are in there on tiny slips of paper and my brother, Darren's, living in Arizona. There's a prayer for Trish, our friend from the health center, whose daughter died of a drug overdose . . . and Nila, my patient who ran away from her husband. Next to it is the prayer candle I light every night. I stop for a moment with my hand on the box, then step out on the porch and smell the fresh-cut grass and something else familiar, wet dirt and growing things.

Here I can look down through the trees at the lights on the other side of Hope Lake, gold streaks on the dark water. I take a deep breath and let it out slowly. It's been a rough few years, but I shouldn't get so freaked out by a phone call. The practice is on solid ground since Dr. Parsons joined. Our three boys are grown and out of college. Two are already fathers.

My secret sadness is that, after thirty years, we no longer deliver babies. I still see patients for early prenatal care, but since the medical malpractice crisis, a few years ago, we gave up our obstetrical liability insurance.

Get over it, girl! I admonish myself. *You're still caring for mothers and teens and red-hot mamas sweltering through menopause.* I lean my arms on the porch rail, staring across the dark water, remembering another phone call twenty years ago.

❦

"It's for you," the ward secretary chirps as she holds out the black receiver. I'm working the 3–11 shift in labor and delivery as an RN at a little hospital north of Columbus. Tom, who after becoming a paramedic had switched to pre-med, was at home with the kids studying bio-chem.

Unusual, I think, *to get a personal call at work. I hope one of the boys isn't sick.*

"Patsy Harman, RN. Can I help you?"

"This is Monica Stewart, coordinator of the University of Minnesota Nurse-Midwifery Program. How are you?"

My heart does a flop. "Fine, thank you." I'd applied to their program six months ago and been put on the wait list, thirteenth in the queue, not an auspicious number. I'm wondering how and why she tracked me down. The program only takes ten students, so Tom and I figured I'd be admitted next year.

"Well, I'll get right to the point," Ms. Stewart goes on. "A student that was supposed to begin our midwifery program had to defer. I'm going through the applications and I wonder if you'd be interested in starting this September."

"This September?"

"Yes. Three weeks. I know it's short notice . . ."

I get it now. Most applicants on the wait list couldn't just pick up and leave, so she's down to me.

"There'd be a small graduate stipend, and we have money for scholarships from the NIH."

"I'd have to get student loans. We don't have any savings. Could I do that in time?"

"We could defer payment until your federal student aid came through."

"OK."

"OK? Don't you need time to think about it? Ask your husband?"

"No. This is what I want to do. This is all I want to do . . ."

For the next hour, while I take care of one labor patient and two postpartum moms, I float two inches above the linoleum floor of the Birthing Suite, waiting to call Tom at break. Finally I get back to a phone.

"Guess what? The University of Minnesota called. They want me to start the midwifery program in three weeks. Someone dropped out and no one wants her spot. They got clear down to number thirteen."

"Lucky thirteen. That's great, Pats."

"You don't mind? I said yes, but it's so soon. We'd have to get up there and find jobs and a place to live . . ."

"We can do it. What's that to all the other things that we've done?"

᙮

Funny how things work out. I release a long sigh, still staring down at Hope Lake, then bend my head back to look at the stars. There's the

Big Dipper, Orion's Belt, the Seven Sisters, the tiny lights that have guided me since I was twenty. A falling star catches my eye and I reach my hands wide . . . then bring them together in a wordless prayer. *Thank you.*

Refuge

"Whoa, did you see that?" Tom's leaning over the porch, pointing down into the woods. After three days of slashing rain, the tail of another Gulf hurricane is gone and we're sitting on the porch of our cedar-sided home, looking down at the lake, enjoying the smells and the sights of our three acres of grass, gardens, and woods. Innocent, small white cumulus clouds, the kind you might see on a postcard, dot the blue sky.

This is our worship, on Sunday mornings, a time of ease and private reflection, a day to make love, to heal, to play music together, to walk in the woods and work in the garden. Well, it *was* private, until Zen, our youngest son, came home a week ago and parked his battered gray Toyota pickup, crammed with all his worldly possessions, in the drive. It's temporary, he tells us. He and his love of the last five years have separated and he's come home to get his head together. *My words, not his.*

I remember how it hurt to leave Stacy, tore something out of me, though I knew it was the right thing to do. Whether you're married or not, for whatever reason, to separate is so painful. In many cases you lose not just your lover, but also your best friend.

"Shit. Did you see?" Tom exclaims. "A *big* bird. I mean really big! It just flew across the cove, over by the cottages where the ducks and crows are raising a racket."

"Maybe it's a hawk."

"No, bigger than that. A buzzard, maybe. I'm going to get the binoculars." My husband, still wearing his plaid flannel pajama bottoms and a *South Park* T-shirt, steps back through the glass bedroom door and returns with two pairs and our well-used *Peterson Field Guide to Birds*. He rests his wire-rim glasses on the rail and adjusts the focus.

The large-winged creature with a white head swoops through the bare branches once more. I look at Tom with big eyes. "An eagle?" We both follow the flight pattern as the wild mallards and tame white ducks that overwinter in the cove amplify a cry of alarm.

The raptor lands in an oak on the slope just below the house. I study its outline. Dark body, white head, white-fanned tail feathers; the predator hunches over, securing its catch with its talons. "A bald eagle!" I whisper. "But eagles don't live here. Maybe higher in the mountains but never here. Do you think it was driven in by the storm?"

Tom doesn't answer. "What's it eating?" he asks in an undertone. Though we're one hundred feet away, we're afraid of spooking the wildlife. Even our movements are careful and muted.

"A fish?"

"No, it's a *duck*. The eagle is eating one of the ducks!" I'm trying to adjust the new binoculars my husband gave me for my birthday. "I can see the yellow bill, and the duck's still alive!"

We've never before, in fifteen years at Hope Lake, seen eagles. The top of the avian food chain has been the red-tailed hawk, and I wonder at this shift in the ecosystem.

The climate is changing. One-hundred-thousand-year-old ice caps are melting. The ocean temperature's rising. Why shouldn't there be an alteration in the bird life in West Virginia? I scan the cottages on the other side of the cove. No one else stands on his or her porch with his or her mouth open. They must be at church.

"Should I call Zen to come see?" I ask Tom.

"Nah, let him sleep."

For twenty minutes we lean on the porch rail, witnessing this biological event. The crows and the ducks continue their warnings. The oaks and the maples say nothing.

☙

I could never stand people who stay in bed all day, even as a hippie. It depresses me. No matter what, I bounce out of bed. There's too much to see, too much to do. I should have used the eagle sighting as an excuse to wake our son. Now the bird's gone . . .

I'm wiping the kitchen counter and Tom's making lunch, grilled cheese sandwiches on sourdough bread, when I hear the clump, clump,

clump of Zen's size-thirteen bare feet coming up the stairs from his bedroom on the lower level. His dark, short straight hair sticks up like he's been on a two-day bender. He pours himself a cup of black coffee.

"I think I was better off when I was living with Callie," Zen finally announces with a long mournful sigh.

In homes all over the U.S., golf course mansions and walk-up apartments, young men and women are returning to their parents' homes when their relationships fall apart, they lose their jobs, or run out of money. Tom and I had prided ourselves that *our boys,* at least, had finished college and were out earning their way. Now Zen comes home, three pairs of his athletic shoes are scattered on the floor of the front hall, every cupboard door is open in the kitchen, and I can't walk around in my underwear anymore.

"You were better off when you lived together?" I ask, like a shrink, not knowing what else to say.

"Yeah. Here at home, I regress, fall into a black pit."

"Maybe you should go back to her," my husband offers. "Maybe you could still make a go of it." Both Tom and I admire Callie, a grad student in environmental engineering at Yale.

"I don't *want* to go back. I love her, but I was just spinning my wheels in New Haven. I couldn't find work, all I had were a few jobs in Web site design. Not enough to make a living, and anyway, I don't really like sitting at a computer all day. We both agree. I need to find a sense of direction."

The three of us sit down at the table and reach for each other's hands, the same way we've done for so many years. My moment of silence is filled with hope and regret. I had thought, after almost ten years of worry, that our boys were settled in adult life, two of them with children of their own, all of them out of college. Now Zen is home again, and I wonder if we've set our children's ideals too high and if that golden bar makes it hard for them.

Love should be passionate and forever! Sex should be ecstatic! Work should be rewarding and fun. Your life should contribute to the greater good and be socially constructive. But there's more . . .

Deer should walk through your yard and eagles fly through the trees below your house. If you choose to have children, they should be happy and healthy and free from fear . . . Trouble is, I still aspire to those things myself.

We squeeze hands at the end of our silent prayer and I break into the Johnny Appleseed song. *The Lord's been good to me. And so I thank the Lord, for giving me the things I need, the rain and the sun and the apple trees . . .*

"Love you guys," Zen says, and he lights the table with a wide grin just like Tom's. Handsome and intelligent, wounded and uncertain, he is home. He is our boy.

HOPE

At noon, I rest my elbows on the conference room table of the women's clinic, thinking about my last patient. I'd spent longer with her than I meant to, but once she started talking, I couldn't move. This happens a lot. The women tell me their stories as they sit in my little exam room on the end of the table in their thin blue cotton exam gowns, and I am spellbound. Carissa had attempted a homebirth and things hadn't gone well. She'd been transferred to the hospital for an emergency C-section. The baby lived, but she still has nightmares. Birth trauma can happen to both women and men, and it will take Carissa a long time to heal. The experience of childbirth is so important. Whether it's wonderful or horrible, the memory imprints.

We are just wrapping up our monthly meeting for the secretarial staff in which we go over ideas to make our office run more smoothly. Tom rarely comes. He leaves the clinic administration to me, having had more meetings than he could stand during our commune days.

"So . . ." says Linda, our vivacious blond receptionist, leaning forward in her chair. She's the practical joker who slaps stickers on your back that say KICK ME and she loves to get me going. All six of the staff look up.

"So . . . tell us about the first delivery you ever did, Patsy. Back in the hippie days . . . The one that got you started."

I smile. "I already told you . . ."

"Not the new people. We have the time."

I replace my apple core in my lunch bag. "You sure?" Everyone nods. They're still munching their french fries.

"Well, this is interesting. I was just talking about that delivery with Tom a few nights ago. We were living on the commune back then, remember, and I was teaching childbirth classes in Spencer.

"I guess you know that in those days, going to the hospital to have your baby was pretty brutal. All women were literally strapped down, given a spinal or saddle block, and delivered with forceps. The fathers weren't allowed in the delivery room and the babies were taken away. You didn't even get to touch them."

"Really?" "No!" "That's awful." These young women in their twenties and thirties are shocked.

"I'm just telling you this to give you some background. Actually, the first birth I did was an accident. Tom was there, but he wasn't a doctor or even a paramedic yet.

"This one evening I went to Laura and Lou's farm out in the country to do one more class. Tom and Mica came, too. When I asked Tom what he remembered about the birth, I was surprised how little he could recall. He mostly remembered the barn they lived in."

"Come on! They lived in a barn . . . like a *manger?*" That's Linda, the smart aleck.

"No, a really cool, converted, insulated barn. Tom reminded me what it looked like. The whole middle space was empty, with a beautiful kitchen. He could even describe the gas stove, an old-fashioned green enameled affair. Have you ever seen one?" Some of the women nod. "We just had a cast-iron woodstove on our commune . . .

"There was also a library and a sitting room and upstairs around the balcony, bedrooms and bathrooms for the four couples and their kids. Above it all, in the center of the structure, and this is the part that Tom loved, there was a white parachute hanging like a canopy. I had forgotten all this, but he could describe it in detail.

"That night, a spring snowstorm came up, covering the ground and making their dirt road too slick to get out, so we slept over. About ten, we went to bed in a spare bedroom upstairs. I woke in the middle of the night with tapping on the door . . .

"One of the women from the commune, Star was her name, stood there with a kerosene lantern, her long yellow hair shining like a halo. 'Can you come, Patsy? Can you come see Laura? Something's going on. She says the baby's coming.'

"I crawled out of the covers, not wanting to wake Mica or Tom, but I shouldn't have worried, they both sleep like logs. I pulled on my jeans and T-shirt and followed her up the stairs.

"At the end of the hall, candlelight flickers from an open doorway and I can hear moaning. *Holy shit!* I think. This sounds like the real thing! Music plays on the stereo, something sweet and mellow with violins.

"When I step into the room, there's Laura, naked on her hands and knees, her dark hair hanging down and her white butt wagging back and forth.

"'Oh, Patsy,' she says. 'Help me!'

"Like, what was I going to do? I'd only seen three babies born, and one was Mica, in a mirror. Lou, the husband, a guy with a long ponytail, filled me in. 'Laura's been having back pain all night, Patsy. We didn't realize it was labor until she felt the urge to push. I just can't believe this. I thought we'd see a bloody show or something! We planned a homebirth and I was supposed to deliver. But I can't. Just look at me, I'm a wreck.' He holds out his trembling hands.

"I lean down to get a better view of Laura's bottom and there's something weird and shiny showing at her vagina.

"'Do you have exam gloves or something, Lou? A birth kit?'" He looks around wildly.

"'Top drawer, bureau . . . ' That was Laura. Despite her moaning and panting she's still got it together. Better than Lou does, that's for sure."

The women around the table are rapt.

"Well, I didn't really know what I was doing, but I had to find out if the baby was at least head down, otherwise we were in deep doo-doo. It was an hour to the nearest hospital, even without the snow.

"So I checked. Turns out, the shiny thing at the opening was the intact amniotic sac. I'd never seen one before. It looks like a silver water balloon.

"I pull on a pair of gloves and stick my fingers in there to feel for the presenting part and the water bag pops. Amniotic fluid squirts all over the place and the hairy little head slides down an inch. This kid is coming, ready or not!

"'Go get Tom, Star!'" I order.

"Tom wanders in. You know him; he never hurries. At a glance he sees what's happening and without any instruction lays the birth stuff out on a baby blanket and puts on gloves.

"'Shit!' Laura growls. 'My back hurts so bad, like nails stabbing into me.' A little poop comes out as the head moves down and Tom wipes it up."

Janie, the youngest of the staff, winces. She's the only one that hasn't given birth and may not know this is common.

"The baby was posterior," I explain to the women. "Sunny-side up. That's what usually causes severe back labor, and women in second stage often have a little bowel movement when the baby's head compresses the rectum."

"So what happened next?" Janie asks.

"Well, I didn't know what I was doing, remember? I'd never delivered a baby before, so I just held on to Laura's bottom to give support.

"She growled like a water buffalo, and slowly the baby's head emerged, the dark hair, then the eyes, then the nose, then the whole body. The baby cried right away, thank God. Everyone was laughing.

"'It's Hope,' Lou said. 'I knew it was a girl.'

"When I looked behind me, the whole commune was standing in the doorway, in the golden candlelight, like angels. That birth changed my life. I'd found my calling."

CHAPTER 2

Lost

"What should I do with my life, Mom?"

After a week in New York City, looking for interesting work and visiting his older brother and his family, Zen is back home again. Neither Mica, an investment consultant, nor his wife, Emma, a reporter, knew of any jobs. For the past two days Zen has prowled the house, lost. He stays up until three and then wakes at noon. I've given up on nagging him.

His question about what he should do with his life takes me aback. I'm usually so full of motherly advice. The one time I'm asked, I go blank. I finish rinsing the stainless steel sink before I speak.

"You OK? I know it's a hard time for you."

"Yeah, I'm fine. I cried a lot today though." He flashes a half smile, carries one of Tom's hand-thrown pottery coffee mugs into the living room, and plops his narrow, six-foot-three body on the blue and mauve upholstered pine factory sofa. I follow with a cup of peppermint tea.

"It's good to cry sometimes." My son doesn't shed tears easily and I can tell by his revelation that he wants to talk.

I rest my feet up on the sturdy wooden coffee table and study his face, the clear skin, high cheekbones, and gray eyes. A good-looking young man, but the gray eyes are sad. His hair is short now and sticks up at the crown.

"I went up to the state park this morning and walked in the woods all the way to the cliffs. You know, where you can see for miles and hear the river roaring below? I could do *anything* with my life. I'm smart enough, and creative." He gives me a sideways glance, grinning at his immodesty, and goes on. "I could be an architect, a photographer, a physician."

Zen is the most intellectually complex of my boys. I catch Van Morrison singing on the stereo, a good song for him. *Searching for the philosopher's stone.*

"You'll figure something out. I didn't go back to school to be a nurse-midwife until I was thirty-two . . ."

Tom interrupts this mother-and-son conversation when he sticks his head in the front door dressed in his white bee suit. "You ready?"

Zen jerks to his feet. "Got to go, Mom."

Prayer

Father and son are off to tend our beehives. We have five on our property, positioned on a platform on the hillside below the garden, and ten others on two nearby farms. I pull on my worn running shoes with the one broken lace; time for me to get to work too. My task this weekend is the garden.

In the garage, I assemble my tools and load the plants in the old red wheelbarrow. By the calendar, it's too early to put in tomatoes, but it's been a very warm spring. I'll take a chance. For two hours, I dig holes with a spade, then crawl along the rows, gently placing the seedlings and tucking them in like their earth mama.

This is work that I can do without thinking. Sometimes, with my hands in the dirt, I feel like the young woman in Minnesota, planting potatoes for the long winter, and then I look up and see the gazebo and realize I live in Blue Rock Estates, a gated lakeside development of mansions and condos and more ordinary contemporary houses like ours.

How many years have Tom and I participated in this yearly sowing and gathering? You turn over the dense and stubborn soil, enrich it with compost, drop in the seeds, and wait for their tiny green leaves to emerge. You water. You weed.

You protect the plants from bugs, birds, and deer. We could purchase packaged vegetables in a supermarket much easier, but this is our link to the days when we believed we could change the world. This is a prayer, a strange way of hoping.

My mind drifts to my coming excursion to New York City with Mara. Tom has to be on call, so I was thrilled when my old friend, who now teaches women's studies in Maryland, agreed to join me on this trip to visit Mica and Emma and their new daughter, Rose. It's been four months since I held the baby.

When I stand to stretch, I'm surprised to see the men already returning in Zen's sputtering pickup. They get out wearing white cotton coveralls and their beekeepers' hats, veils, and gloves, and walk stiffly toward the garden like scientists from the CDC protected from deadly viruses. Tom carries a beekeeper's bellow that belches foul smoke. Zen has an armful of hive tools.

"We finished the Johnsons' farm," my husband reports, his face creased with worry behind the bee veil. "They look weak, and I don't know why. Four of the hives are completely dead. It's a bad scene. I fed them sugar water for a month this spring and I medicated them for mites, but they aren't making brood like they should be and I can't find one of the queens. It might be that colony collapse disorder that's happening all over the country. We're going to work on the hives below the garden now." Father and son disappear behind the forsythia bushes, two men, careful in their work, moving gently among the potentially dangerous insects.

Maybe Zen should be a professional beekeeper, I consider. Now there's an idea! Wild bees are almost nonexistent in the United States . . . If it weren't for people like my husband, fussing over the domestic ones, few plants could pollinate. Bees are more important than animals in terms of human survival. If bees were to disappear, plants couldn't propagate and human life would soon flicker out. I sit back on my knees and gaze at our fruit trees, their blossoms already setting small peaches.

The sun is just dipping below the horizon when the three of us finish our chores and lie down in the grass. The sun drifts lower and drops crimson behind the mountains. I let out a long sigh, feel the earth beneath me, and reach for Tom's wide hand on one side and Zen's long thin hand on the other.

ZEN

The feeling of the earth under me is always healing. The day I went into labor with Zen, I lay on the grass with Tom, just like this, and the earth gave me peace that day too.

☙

It's February 13, a warm shirtsleeve day in Spencer. Above us, bare branches net the sun.

Contractions are every twelve minutes. As usual I was a few weeks past my due date, a few weeks or a few days, I never knew because my periods were so irregular and we didn't have ultrasounds then. Or maybe they had them in the big cities, but not in Roane Country.

"Do you think we called the midwives too early? This could be false labor. I'm not leaking fluid. What if they drive all this way and nothing happens?" Tom puts his arm around me.

"Come on, Pats. They live in Athens, two hours away. It's your *third* baby. You might go fast."

"Right!" This is uttered with sarcasm. "Mica took *twenty-four hours*. Orion took *fifteen*." I massage my belly as another contraction comes on.

"Mmmf. They *are* picking up though. Let's keep walking." Tom helps me up and once again we march around the block, humming John Philip Sousa's "Stars and Stripes Forever." Uphill and down we march, around and around, until we get back to the Gray House, a little bungalow we're renting in town while I attend Arch Moore Vocational to become an LPN. Mica is with my two women friends from school, Tara and Kris, the only other hippie chicks in the program. Orion is with Mara at her place.

Alone in the two-bedroom cottage, Tom and I make love. Not our most romantic. I'm in a get-it-done mood. Then he helps me with an enema, thinking it will increase the contractions. Neither of us have ever done this before, and we're laughing so hard, I almost don't make it to the toilet. By the time my midwives, Lucy and Clo, arrive, it's getting dark and my cervix is five centimeters dilated.

The labor creeps on while James Taylor sings on our little boom box. Tom and I slow dance, while the birth attendants sip herbal tea in the kitchen and carefully monitor the sound of my voice. *When the pitch goes up, they'll know I'm seven or eight centimeters. When it drops, I'm ready to push.*

For the first time, I realize what I need to do to make the contractions more effective and less painful is just sink down on them. I bounce with my knees and they don't hurt as much. Though I've coached scores of women through labor, this is a revelation.

Around eleven, I get cranky and stomp into the bedroom. "I'm sick of *Steamroller Blues!* I'm tired and I wish everyone would go home!"

Lucy realizes without checking me that I'm in transition. "We're calling in the troops," she announces and gets on the phone. "Put some hot water on and lay the birth stuff out." By the time Tara and Kris show up with Mica and, a few minutes later, Mara arrives with Orion, Zen's head is almost crowning.

This time I'm not pushing the baby out; it's pushing me. No slow buildup like a freight train getting started . . . I'm skidding along the tracks in front of the cowcatcher.

When I open my eyes during a contraction, I see Orion and Mica, holding on to each other, at the end of the bed, in a circle of candle- light. They look so worried I stop midpush. "It's OK," I reassure them. "Mama's just working hard."

Tom sits behind me, holding me up, and, for a change, lets the midwife catch. When Zen emerges, three minutes after midnight on St. Valentine's Day, he greets the world with a long trembling wail.

"Is he OK? Is he OK?" I ask. It's obvious he is, but as soon as the placenta comes out, I just want to sleep. I've never been like this after a delivery.

"Take my blood pressure, Lucy! I feel weird. Something must be wrong."

"Nope, you're fine . . . one twenty over eighty."

"I'm shaking so hard, I feel like I've been run over. I just want to close my eyes and shut everything out."

"So, sleep," she says. "We'll give you some space. Tom's got the baby. It's Zen, right? That's his name?" They all withdraw into the kitchen and I pull a blanket over my head. It's not that I'm so tired. I'm just so shaken by the power of the birth.

In twenty minutes I'm myself again when little Orion toddles into the bedroom carrying the birthday cake and almost drops it on me.

Happy Birthday to you. Happy Birthday dear Zen, we sing, and we are all so happy to have this new life.

⚜

A breeze comes up and showers peach blossoms down on us. "Hey," I laugh, holding my hands up into them. Zen, now a man, rests with Tom and me on the lawn, looking down at Hope Lake. I ask the green grass to enter his head, bring peace to his tangled brain.

Voices

It's nearing midnight when the shadow of the Appalachian Ridge rises up in the distance like a great sleeping bear. My weekend in New York City wasn't the easygoing visit with Mica and his family I expected. The first thing that happened was that Mica announced that he, Emma, and their baby, Anna, are moving to Moscow for five years. Emma has been offered her dream job as a foreign correspondent, and Mica has always been interested in living abroad. *But Moscow, shit, that's half a world away.* I felt like crying, but I kept it together. Now my traveling companion and I are on our way home.

"Thanks for being my navigator, Mara. You're better at *navigating* and better at soothing my grandbaby. You're more gracious than I am, sing tighter harmony, and keep up a more stimulating conversation. You're even better at mothering my son than I am."

"What?"

"When we said good-bye to Mica, you looked up in his eyes, held his shoulders, and said, 'I'm so *proud* of you.' He needs to hear that from *me.* I don't know when I last told him that. I was too freaked out that they are moving to Moscow to say something supportive. What *I* said was

'Do you think you'll be able to find a job there?' What's he going to do while Emma works as a reporter?"

Mara, still married to Benny and now mother of her own three grown kids, reaches over and pats my leg comfortingly. "Thanks for the compliment, even if it's not true, but you're so *brave* and I'm so timid. If it hadn't been for your invitation, I'd have never gotten to New York City."

"Brave?" I repeat. "I don't think of myself as brave. I'm Chicken Little! . . . You'd think at my age I'd have everything figured out, but I don't have a clue and I'm more confused than when I was thirty."

"Oh, come on."

"No, really, get this. The other day, I was out in the driveway spraying the weeds in the cracks with Roundup, and at the same time pondering how we could get a wind generator to harness the energy of the wind off the lake. Then it strikes me. *Get a grip, girl!* You're spraying the earth with a powerful toxin! I had to laugh.

"It humbled me. How different are Tom and I from the average American? We used to try so hard to be socially and environmentally responsible. Nothing has changed in the world, except the things we tried to warn people about thirty years ago are now coming true." I fade off, staring at the highway where it drops into the night.

Thirty years. Has it really been that long?

"Do you think we can make it, Mara? I mean, the planet. Things are changing so fast. It seems out of control. The climate is erratic . . . the atmosphere's heating up. It's a house of cards that could go down fast. What kind of world are we going to leave for our children and grandchildren?"

Mara gives me a nudge and silently points to a deer on the side of the road. *I'd better slow down. Hitting a deer is not a small accident.*

I think of my boys as we wind through the cut at Sideling Hill and speed past the Hazelton prison, all lit up like a fairy castle. Zen is in Maui with a friend, Joplin. It isn't a solution to what he should do with his life, but at least he's doing *something*.

Orion is being a home daddy to his seven-month-old baby boy and the five-year-old stepdaughter he loves like his own, still doing his art, but as his drawings become more tender and refined, he gets more discouraged. Employment teaching art at the university level is hard to find. Let's face it, employment of any kind, lately, is hard to find.

And Mica and Emma are getting ready for their five-year sojourn in Moscow! I recall my own mother, how easily I left her to go hitchhiking around the country; I barely gave a thought to how she might feel, not seeing me, or her grandsons, but once or twice a year. Now my heart twists for her.

♃

Mara has fallen asleep, her head against the passenger window, so I turn on the radio, hoping the music will keep me awake. Leonard Cohen is singing "Hallelujah." I first heard the song at Chester Creek House when I was twenty-seven. Jim played it over and over. The faces of those days recede, but the melody is part of me. The song is so beautiful and sad, the way life is, the way it seems when you're older.

Sounds of Silence

Sometimes you can see trouble coming like a line of dark clouds on the horizon, moving over the mountains. Other times, trouble comes like a flash flood; suddenly the gulley fills with a torrent of muddy water and you're flattened against the rocks.

♃

Saturday, while Tom and I are playing a duet, a minuet in G major by Bach, on the piano and string bass, the phone rings.

It's Mica, and he starts off with an expression of guilt about not calling. We put him on speakerphone.

"I'm sorry I haven't phoned or e-mailed. It's just been so hectic here arranging to ship our stuff to Moscow and also, you know how I am, I didn't want to say anything until I had the full story, but I guess you better get out another candle, Mom . . ." *I go very still.* The little votive that I light every night sits right by my prayer box.

Tom doesn't react one way or another. He's slumped on the sofa, staring straight ahead, with his hairy legs and wide, bare hobbit feet on the coffee table.

"You know how Rose didn't pass her hearing screen when we left labor and delivery? The postpartum nurse said maybe her ear canals were still too little and to wait and have her examined later?"

"I remember," I cut in. "But so what? We didn't even have hearing tests when we gave birth to you guys."

"Well, we didn't go for a recheck right away because she seemed fine, reacted to what we said and everything, but last week we finally decided we'd better get it done before we moved." Here his voice breaks. "And they think Rose can't hear."

Tom and I sit in shock. Except for the bubbler in the fish tank, there's no sound. Mica goes on.

"What the doctors say is, they think she has a congenital inner-ear defect called bilateral atresia, closed canals, and what's worse, it can be associated with terminal disorders of the kidneys and the heart, even Lou Gehrig's disease and muscular dystrophy." The living room walls close around me.

"Have you gotten a second opinion?" I finally break in.

"We're trying to. It takes weeks to get an appointment with a specialist at Columbia Presbyterian Hospital."

I try to restore hope. "When I was there she seemed *perfect* to me, alert and responsive. I can't believe she doesn't hear. Remember when I sang to her in the rocker and she fell asleep? I'm *sure* she heard me."

Am I really sure? Or was it the rhythmic motion of the rocking chair and the vibrations that came from my chest?

We hang up, and without saying anything head for the bedroom. Tom flops down on the bed. The smell of blooming locust trees comes in through the open door. With a heavy heart, I light my prayer candle and squirm into my husband's strong arms.

I want him to make everything better. He kisses my neck, pulls me against his chest, and *does* make things better, at least for this night.

Lullaby

The medical information about Rose's condition dribbles in over the next few weeks. First the results of the ultrasounds. No heart defects. No kidney defects. All the baby's vital systems are fine, but with each specialist appointment there *is* consensus: Rose's ears are perfect on the outside, but the eustachian tubes are closed. She does, indeed, have bilateral atresia. We've never had a baby born with a physical disability in our family. Why did I think we were immune?

I rest back in one of the white canvas chairs that face the corner living room windows. I've been so worried that something terminal was wrong with Rose that her being hearing impaired no longer seems terrible. Outside, the peach, pear, and apple trees are showing green lumps of fruit and the Shasta daisies are blooming.

My mother-heart is scared to death for Rose . . . but my midwife-heart says, *Hold on! Rose doesn't know that there's anything wrong with her. She's happy, clean, breastfed, and loved. Watch. Wait. God will be with us.*

Good news comes when we learn that the audiologists believe that Rose may have only an 85 percent hearing loss, so her inner ear, the part that connects to the brain, is intact. If they're correct, then Rose can be fitted with a tiny bone-conduction hearing aid, and when she's five or six she may be eligible for surgery. The genetic test to determine if Rose is at risk for more lethal defects takes the longest to come back. I finally have to ask Mica over the phone.

"Shit, I forgot to tell you!" he explodes. "We were going to cancel the move to Russia if Rose had serious medical problems, but once we got the word that she's genetically normal, it's full speed ahead. We've been working like crazy to get ready. I never knew what a hassle it was to get visas."

"So . . . ? What did the geneticist *say?*"

"Well, Rose is just a normal little girl with blind ear pouches, and we're getting a bone-conduction hearing aid before we leave."

*

On Friday, I arrange to record, at a small studio on the edge of town, a CD of lullabies for Rose, so she can hear me sing when she gets her hearing aid. I'll have copies made for Orion's kids too, Lissic and Abraham.

At first my voice is weak, but I don't let myself cry, neither for joy or sadness. I close my eyes and pretend I'm singing in the dark to Mica, Orion, and Zen when they were little boys, and my voice gets stronger. *Hush-a-bye don't you cry. Go to sleep-y little baby* . . .

CHAPTER 3

Healer

"What's up?" I ask as I come out through the open deck door.

Tom sits with his feet up on the porch rail, staring across the lawn. "I'm just waiting for a call. A patient I did surgery on a few days ago came back to the emergency room this evening." Two gray squirrels with curly tails are eating birdseed spilled by the careless blue jays, two feet away from his chair, but he doesn't notice.

His cell phone finally rings and he flips it open. "Dr. Harman." I listen to the one-sided conversation, watching his face. There are circles under his eyes. He's been harassed with phone calls two nights in a row. "Yeah, so how are her vitals? . . . OK, wait for the lab results. Type and cross her for two units and make her NPO."

"What?" I ask when he hangs up.

"I've got to go back to the hospital." His voice is low and discouraged.

I tighten my lips. "Can't you eat dinner first?"

"It's my patient Bobbie Boyd. The RN says she's orthostatic, blood pressure's way too low."

"Is she bleeding?"

"Not on the outside, but she oozed all through surgery. I ordered a post-op hemoglobin and blood-clotting studies. They're pending. I guess I can grab a bite."

Five minutes later, his cell phone rings again, a catchy salsa tune that belies my foreboding.

"Dr. Harman," he says again. "I'll be right there. Call the nursing supervisor and alert the OR."

"What's happening?"

"Her hemoglobin is 6."

He doesn't have to say more. Six is way too low, and he's already heading toward the front door.

❦

It's a warm evening, and I'm outside in the gazebo staring down at the lake. The air smells like lilacs, and even if I was blind, I could tell by the scent that it's almost summer. The fireflies come out one by one, the first I've seen this year, but I don't get as excited as usual. Tom's still not home.

Because of his specialty, pelvic pain, my husband takes care of many women who've been referred to him by other gynecologists, surgeons, and family docs, women with endometriosis and adhesions, women in delicate health or with autoimmune diseases that lead to poor healing, patients the other docs prefer not to mess with. Tom always accepts them.

I think of the worst: what if Bobbie Boyd hemorrhaged and died? Tom's never had a woman expire after surgery or childbirth and I don't know how he'd handle it.

Finally, the lights of the 4Runner come down the drive. "Tom, out here . . ." I call across the lawn. "How'd you do? She OK?"

My husband sags into the deck chair next to me. "Yeah . . ."

I think that's all he's going to say and I'm afraid to ask more.

"We had to give her another two units of blood, four all together. By the time I opened her, I couldn't find a bleeder, but there was one thousand ccs in her pelvis." I picture the amount as almost a quart. "Her labs showed a coagulation disorder. I stayed a few hours longer to be sure she was OK, but her husband was pissed."

I imagine the man, skinny and tall, with a scraggly ponytail, wearing a tight AC/DC T-shirt. He sits on the edge of the hospital bed, tightens his jaw, gets out a pack of cigarettes, and then remembers he's in a hospital and puts them back. When Dr. Harman comes in, weary and wearing light green scrubs, the fellow jumps up. "What did you do to her? Will she be OK? She better be OK."

"The vibes were heavy," Tom continues, discouraged. "The guy's an asshole. I've seen the way he treats Bobbie when he brings her to the clinic. He talks *for her,* bosses her around like she's a piece of shit. I don't think he trusts me."

I stand up behind my husband's chair and run my fingers through his short gray hair and across his forehead, pull his head back until it rests on my stomach. He's such a good man.

It once seemed so easy. We wore our hearts on our sleeves and were here to serve the people, first by attending homebirths when there were no birthing centers or hospitals with humane protocols, and later as medical professionals who changed those protocols.

When Laurel left the commune, Tom was my driver as we sped through the night to homebirths, down a hollow or on the top of a mountain. He boiled water and sat in the kitchen. The fathers appreciated having another man around, a reassuring presence in a sea of femaleness. I appreciated him because he was an EMT and available if we had an emergency.

Now he is the captain of the ship, the one in charge, losing sleep over surgical complications and worries about malpractice litigation. When we step out of the gazebo and look up, heavy clouds have come in and the stars are wiped out.

Summer

CHAPTER 4

Escape

"You gonna be ready soon?" I pester, standing at the door to my husband's pottery studio, inhaling the earthy smell of clay.

"Bug off, Pats." Tom is hunched over a table covered with pale gray vessels, mostly coffee mugs, and he's not in the mood for my comments. The floor is sprayed with clay; even the windows are splattered. His glazed bowls, pitchers, teapots, and vases, in shades of blue, brown, and green, cover every surface of every shelf lining the walls.

"Gotta move if we're going to make the ferry," I nag.

"I have to get the handles on these mugs while the clay is still damp. There's plenty of time."

I let out a long sigh, then stomp back upstairs to my office. It won't help to push him. He only gets more stubborn. We take turns alternating who will be worried about being late. Apparently, this is my turn.

On my silver laptop, a recent e-mail from Laurel is open. I run my fingers lightly over the screen. Our old commune friend is always sending some political announcement, some call to action or silly YouTube video. I forward the best ones on to Mara and Tom. It's been two years since I've seen Laurel. Maybe three. She's a physical therapist now, married to another physical therapist in Ohio, and has two kids.

"Mica, Emma, and baby Rose are moving to Russia," I type back. "I *hate* that they will be so far away. I'm trying to be brave, but it feels like a chunk of my heart was cut out."

Laurel, having been Mica's stepmom, still asks about the little blond, blue-eyed hippie boy. She has teens of her own, with all the troubles I once had. Recently she e-mailed that she found marijuana in the oldest girl's bureau. *Been there. Done that. The mother-heart drops down a dark hole . . .*

You raise your kids with respect; teach them to think for themselves. You do your best and then they go wild on you. Though all of us were at least peripherally involved with grass in our youth, drugs are much stronger now and more dangerous, not to mention still illegal in most places.

I glance again at my watch, send my e-mail, and snap my laptop closed. This afternoon we're leaving for a long weekend at our summer cottage, Harmony House, a five-bedroom yellow farmhouse with a barn on Pelee Island. The small landmass, about the size of Manhattan but with only three hundred year-round residents, is located on the Canadian side of Lake Erie.

I laugh at myself. Once we lived in a log cabin, before that a barn with a dirt floor, then there was the butterfly tent. What yuppies we are, with two lakeside homes! I wait twenty minutes, then bug Tom again.

❦

Four hours later, just in time, we trot up the ramp of the old-fashioned red and white ferry. As the copper sun drops over the edge of the earth, we pull, with three long, low blasts of a horn, out of Sandusky Bay.

Tom and I stand on the bow watching white sailboats pass in the dusk. "I'm so tense lately." I let out my shaky air, indicating with my fist my upper abdomen. "Too tense." Tom's elbows rest on the deck rail and his face is impassive, but I want to talk.

"For months, when your mom was sick, we had to go back and forth to Ohio. Our life has been in turmoil, and then she dies while you're in the Dominican Republic doing your medical mission, and we go back for the funeral and then Zen comes home and our house isn't ours anymore. Just when things are calming down, Mica announces that they're moving to Moscow and then we find out Rose can't hear. It's like a beehive that won't settle."

Tom puts his arm around me and squeezes but he doesn't say anything, just stares at the swath of red sky turning lavender. A squeal on the bow of the boat interrupts the quiet. The captain, a slim man with short white hair, wearing a red plaid kilt and a crisp shirt with gold crests, tunes up his bagpipe. He squeezes a few times, then begins a Scottish drone.

Amazing Grace, how sweet the sound . . . the words fill my head. The fist in the center of my abdomen opens. *That saved a wretch like me.* I close my eyes and am back in the Spencer Library community room at the Growing Tree potluck supper. We're holding hands in a circle. *I once was lost, but now I'm found* . . .

The tables are laden with hippie food, cornbread, pinto beans, and vegetables from our gardens. Mara is there, and Stacy. Rachel catches my eye. Laurel is leading the singing, with Ben playing his guitar.

I used to think our life on the farm was so hard. Maybe all life is hard. I glance at Tom to see if the bagpipe music moves him too. Our eyes meet and I know he remembers.

The piper plays to the water. He plays to the first star, the one that gave me courage when I lay on the ridge in labor with Orion. He plays for us.

Through many dangers, toils and snares we have already come. 'Tis grace that brought us safe thus far . . .

"Welcome to Canada," a passenger laughs. *And grace will lead us home.*

Regret

In an hour, we're sitting, with a bottle of wine, on our deck, which rests on top of the granite break-wall, protecting our summer home from storms. "Cheers," I say, clinking our glasses. "Happy summer solstice." To the south, on the U.S. shore, twenty miles away, distant lights twinkle in Sandusky and Lorain.

A few years ago, when we were on vacation and feeling flush, before the economy went to hell, we bought this farmhouse with a barn and two acres, and now, to keep up with the mortgage, rent it to cottagers from May to November. We started coming to Pelee when the boys were little and Tom was in medical school in Ohio. We camped here at first, then moved up to cabins. The kids learned to drive on these dirt roads. Below the huge boulders, the waves measure time.

Both of us let out a long breath together. Each August there's more algae bloom and matted weeds as the water temperature rises. I lean forward to look down at the rocky beach and when I rest back, notice Tom's eyes. "Are you OK?"

"Yeah. I was just thinking of my mom. She never got a chance to see this place. Her dying has really hit me. It's been months since her funeral, but every day I think of something I want to tell her. I miss her. She was one of my best friends."

"Are you crying?"

He swipes the eyes with the back of his hand. "A little . . ."

How could I have not noticed? I reach over and touch his wet cheek with one finger, then take him in my arms. Just because Dorothy's death had been anticipated doesn't mean it wasn't traumatic.

Sometimes I wonder about myself, *the sensitive midwife*. Am I so wrapped in my work with women that I don't even notice the pain of my own family members? How often have I walked past Tom or the boys, deep in thought about a patient, completely oblivious to the ones I love most?

"I miss her," my husband says again between sobs. "I miss my mom." His chest shakes against mine. "She was an inspiration to me, even on her deathbed. So strong, facing the unknown. Even when speaking was exhausting, she was herself—demanding, compassionate, sometimes a pain in the ass . . . I just wish I'd been there to say good-bye. I wish I'd stayed home, not gone on that medical mission to the Dominican Republic."

He says that now, but at the time there were nurses, doctors, and impoverished patients needing his care, depending on him. His mother could have lasted for months . . . but she didn't.

❦

It cuts you to see a grown man cry. In thirty years, I can count on one hand the times my husband has broken down. Now I'm crying too. We hold each other with the dark water splashing below.

"Your mama's OK," I tell him, patting his back. "She's probably in heaven dancing with your dad while Bing Crosby sings 'Blue Moon' . . ."

Tom gives me a crooked smile. I pull him up and we slow dance on the deck, like teenagers, our arms locked around each other. *Blue mooooon* . . . . I sing.

"Dancing in heaven?"

"Well, she could be!"

He squeezes me and runs his hands down my back and then lower. Our bodies fit together like an arm in the sleeve of a favorite soft shirt. He kisses me and rubs his two-day beard on my cheek.

It's not easy to let go when you're used to gripping life with your fingernails. It takes a while, but I finally stop struggling, let my wings unfold, and we soar over Lake Erie together.

Ruby Tuesday

My first patient when we get back on Tuesday is Ruby Mott. I think of the Rolling Stones song "Ruby Tuesday" and smile. I'm in a good mood after our mini-vacation and hum a few lines while I look over her chart, then enter the exam room.

"So, Ruby. How's your pain this month?" The twenty-nine-year-old gives me a tired look, as if it's too much to answer. She's a tall, thin woman wearing sandals, fringed jean shorts, and a black tank top. She's so skinny, it crosses my mind that she could have an eating disorder, like Nora, my patient who almost died of bulimia.

Ruby holds her abdomen, looking like death warmed over, and I ask my question again. "So, how's your pain?

"Some days better. Some days worse. I've been under a lot of stress lately."

I hesitate. If I ask about her stress, I may be here for a while. I ask anyway . . . she wants to tell me. "What's up?"

"Money problems. My phone was shut off and my stepmom won't lend me any cash. My dad's in county lockup, so he can't help. I need something for my nerves, can you give me some Valium?"

I frown. This is the kind of social situation a lot of the chronic-pelvic-pain patients have. In-law problems, outlaw problems, kid problems, money problems, yet they faithfully show up, once a month, on Tuesday, for their support group and prescriptions.

I remind myself that women like Ruby are not the average pelvic-pain patients. Most women with endometriosis or lower abdominal adhesions or fibroids or cysts get better with medical therapy or surgery.

The *chronic* pain patients are the hard cases. They've been to multiple doctors looking for help. They've already had several operations, scopes, ablations, nerve blocks, even complete hysterectomies; still they have real pain.

Tom decided on this specialty when he was in his last year of residency. He takes the patients' problems seriously. It's common for women experiencing pain to have been told there's nothing wrong with them . . . that it's all in their heads.

There are some, like Cindy Carlton, who are stable on their meds and never ask for more. Cindy's an elementary school teacher who has massive adhesions from a pelvic infection after surgery years ago. She has two girls and a husband who's a coal miner. One of their kids got married last spring and Cindy brought us pictures of the wedding. The pleasant patient takes narcotics as scheduled. Never asks for more. Without them, she couldn't work, couldn't take care of her family.

If there were an adequate pain center in the area, one that cared about the patients and looked at their problems holistically, we would long ago have referred Cindy and Ruby, but there's nothing like that, so our chronic-pelvic-pain program grows.

"That's tough about the money, Ruby. Maybe you could call the help line at United Way. They might be able to give you a loan." I ignore the request for Valium, but ask her about her BMs, her bladder, her nutrition and activity level. The answers are brief and the appointment comes to an end when I give the young woman her Oxycontin prescription, a handout on stress reduction, and her birth-control pills.

"Thanks, Patsy." The forlorn face breaks into a grin and I watch as she almost skips down the hall and out through the waiting room.

Sometimes I question how much she hurts. Is it all a big show? You hate to second-guess your patients.

No one knows. She comes and goes. Good-bye, Ruby Tuesday.

DESTINY

Sun glints on the river. Blue sky overhead. There's nothing like a free outdoor concert, and these guys are good. The drummer beats out a solo that sounds like a big Harley racing through the mountains and then the band breaks into Bob Seger's "Against the Wind." The crowd cheers, stands up, and sings.

In front of us, a row of men and women tip beers wrapped in paper bags. The lettering on the back of their black T-shirts reads THE PATRIOT GUARD, THE TRIBE OF JUDAH, and THE RIDGE RIDERS. I squeeze my husband's hand, throw my head back, and sing with them . . . *Searching for shelter again and again . . . running against the wind.*

᙮

A woman with big hair walks over, waves a Virginia Slim, and pulls two school-age boys in front of us. "These are the people that helped you get born!" she announces. "My husband, Adam—you remember him, Patsy—is over looking at the BMW power cruisers." The youngsters stare with big brown eyes, embarrassed to be on display.

This happens a few times a week, at the supermarket, the hardware store, or the gas station, to all midwives and OBs. Someone comes up with a toddler or a teen and wants to show us the baby we delivered. It's a small town and I'm glad for the reminders of what we've meant to people.

When the woman drifts off, I whisper to Tom, "Who was *she?*"

"Works in the operating room at the hospital, Brandy something. Used to be at Bargain City, remember? We bought a TV from her once."

I see it now. When the department store went bust and she lost her job, Brandy sat in my exam room crying. I held her hand and wiped her wet cheeks, a single mother in her twenties with a one-year-old I'd delivered, no job and no money. I braided her long hair, as I'd braided it when she was in labor. She took my suggestion and enrolled at the vocational school in the LPN program.

A few years later, Brandy got pregnant a second time and returned to the clinic. This time she held out her left hand to show me a gold wedding band.

❦

"I got married last fall," Brandy says with a grin, "and we ended up preggers a month later. Adam is thrilled. It's his first."

"How'd you meet him?" I ask as I do her new-OB exam.

"Don't laugh . . ."

"I won't!"

"The Internet."

"Lots of my patients have met guys that way. I figure, what the heck, it's worth a try." *The patient doesn't know about my hitchhiking history. Internet dating hardly seems scary.*

Seven months later, Brandy goes into labor. Adam, her husband, a manager at Radio Shack, is with her, and Brandy's mom and her first son, three-year-old Walker. The plan is for Grandma to take the little boy out of the birthing room when the baby comes, but the labor goes so fast and so smoothly he never leaves.

Brandy delivers standing up at the bedside. Tom, stopping by the birthing center on his way from the OR, pours oil over my fingers just like the old days, while I squat behind her on the birthing stool. I can't really see what I'm doing, but I just hold on and the baby slips out.

Little Walker stays right at my side observing everything. He doesn't flinch, doesn't even look frightened. Tom helps him cut his sister's cord, like he once helped Mica. They name the baby Destiny.

❦

The next day, I asked Brandy how she felt about the birth. "Didn't it hurt? You were a lot more emotional at your first delivery."

"No," she told me, her face relaxed and pink. "I wasn't afraid. I had everyone I loved around me, and I had you."

I thought about that. When I was in midwifery school at the university we learned about the factors that affect the progress of labor, the four P's: the *power*—the strength of contractions; the *passenger*—the size and position of the fetus; the *passage*—the shape of the mother's pelvis; and the *psyche*—the mother's state of fear or confidence.

Some childbirth professionals add a fifth P. The *persons* helping you have the baby—competent, caring providers, supportive family and friends or nervous Nellies pacing the floor.

Now that I think of it, you could add a sixth P, *place*. I've always felt that a woman does best in an environment that makes her feel secure. For some, this would be a high-risk hospital, for others a birthing center, for others their home.

❦

As the concert ends, I'm still thinking of Brandy. How many women, like her, have I touched and forgotten? How many have touched me, sisters of mercy?

I imagine their hands carrying me over troubled waters, some calloused from hard labor, some with manicured nails, some with tattoos on the back of their wrists.

CHAPTER 5

Dismissal

"Tom?" I'm standing in the hall that leads to his study, staring at the light that comes under the door. "Are you still up?" I enter without knocking. I thought he'd gone down to Zen's room to sleep. Sometimes he does this when he's restless and has had too much coffee.

My husband sits slumped in his black leather chair wearing brown plaid pajamas with a bright yellow Wild Turkey T-shirt that he got for free when he went to the liquor store. It's a holdover from our hippie trash-picking days. We can't pass up a giveaway. A glass of Wild Turkey sits on his desk. His iPod is plugged into both ears and he's concentrating on a video game.

"Tom!" I say a little louder. He looks up, surprised.

"Don't you have to get up at six thirty?"

"Yeah, what time is it?"

"Three!"

"Shit."

"What's wrong with you, anyway? Haven't you slept at all?"

He kicks the leather footstool toward me and offers me a sip of his drink. "I had to fire a patient today."

"Fire a patient?" I squint, not knowing his meaning.

"Yeah, you know, dismiss her from the practice. Her drug screen was positive for cocaine and negative for her prescription narcotics."

"That means she's not taking the medication you prescribed but *is* snorting coke?"

"Maybe shooting up. Who knows."

"Is she someone I know?"

Tom looks so sad. "Yeah. It's Gladys. She was probably selling her narcotics. The ER docs say you can get fifty dollars each for one of those little 10-milligram pills. Gladys was on three pills daily. That's a hundred and fifty a day. Not bad money, and she probably needs the cash."

My throat tightens. "Gladys is the diabetic, with the boy that they sent to the detention center and the two other younger kids at home?" I want to defend her. "Are you *sure* the test was right? She seemed like such a straight shooter, and she's been our patient for years."

My husband shrugs. "I know . . . and I really liked her. That's what hurts. She'll be calling when she gets the dismissal letter, begging for another chance, but I'm not going to fold. I thought my instincts about people were pretty good. I used to know whom to trust . . . but not now."

"Come on, bud. You got to be in the OR in the morning." My friend lets me lead him to bed.

"Thanks," he says as I tuck him in. No matter how stressed, in two minutes he's snoring. Tonight is no different. The Wild Turkey probably helps.

I stand watching him sleep. He looks smaller tonight, diminished, not the Tom I once knew . . .

CHAPTER 6

Rescue

Toes curled over the wooden edge of our floating dock, I steel myself, then dive deep into Hope Lake, today so clear I can see the sand and pebbles on the bottom. The shock of the cold water makes me want to shout, but I keep my mouth closed and rise, shaking my wet hair, into a world of green. The dark August green of oak leaves, the jungle green of locust, the shamrock green of maple.

I am alone. Tom has gone north to Ohio to meet with his mother's lawyer and settle her estate. I'm hoping it will bring him closure about his mom's death, but not sure it will help. Zen is still out West, surfing, climbing mountains, finding a little work when he can. I smile. Basically living like a hippie.

It's just Roscoe, our beagle-basset, and me left to take care of the gardens and fruit trees. I'll have time to read, to write, to swim, to take a solo bike ride or dance naked to the Grateful Dead in the bedroom if the mood strikes me.

After an hour of letting the silver minnows nibble my toes, I drape my wet towel around my sunburned neck and amble up the wood and stone steps to the house. An alarming buzz, like the sound of a man's electric shaver, catches my attention as I cross the lawn. When I turn toward the hives at the lower edge of the garden, I see thousands of bees shooting up like a Roman candle. I've never seen anything like it and decide that the heat must be making the insects extra frisky.

Inside, as I prepare a dinner of green beans, tomatoes, and squash from the garden, I glance periodically out the windows. Our suburban homestead is growing, two vegetable plots, seven fruit trees, and five hives of bees, but maybe it's getting out of control. *Masses* of bees are now pouring upward, a swirling tornado of insects. What I fear is a swarm.

The phenomenon of a swarm is a natural method of propagation that occurs when a colony gets too crowded; it's good for the bees, bad for the beekeepers. That's why Tom and Zen were moving the bee boxes around a few months ago, making enough room for the brood, checking to see that there was only one queen to each hive.

Apparently they'd missed a queen cell and now she's hatched and is going off on her own. The unfortunate part is, she's taking an army of workers for her new empire, and before the insects abandon ship, they suck up all the honey they can hold. I watch closely the direction of their movements. Higher and higher they rise over the tops of the tallest oaks, their little bodies shining in the evening light. If they escape, they will take all the honey and, as wild bees, never survive the winter.

Ten minutes later, I'm dressed in Tom's white coveralls, complete with gloves, hat, and veil, looking, but not feeling, like a beekeeper. I have no clue what I'm doing, but Tom puts so much time and energy into caring for his hives, I would feel terrible if the swarm got away without me even *trying* to catch them.

I approach the row of forsythia bushes with caution, the Sherlock Holmes of beekeepers. Where would the swarm go? The massive migration has stopped, but a high-pitched drone seems to come from the gazebo. As I move closer, the sound gets louder, until looking up I see, fifteen feet above me, attached to a branch in the peach tree, a lump of bees the size of a beach ball. I've located the renegades; now what? I remember years ago reading a pamphlet about catching a swarm . . . what did it say?

First, find a washtub or a box . . . We don't have a washtub. Maybe a bee box? I truck back to the garage and locate a leftover white wooden beehive with a separate metal cover, then tromp back to the peach tree and place the box under the ball of bees. I'm winging it here, and the light is fading. When night comes, I have no idea what the bees will do. Do they sleep?

The agricultural handout said something about banging a pan to get the bees down . . . What do I have to lose? As fast as I can, in full beekeeper's outfit, I waddle back to the house and grab two stainless steel cooking pots. Bang! Bang! Bang! The bees buzz a little louder, but that's all. *Maybe I can shake them down.*

Tentatively, I take hold of the trunk. Shake. No action. I could climb up the tree and get a better grip on the branch they're hanging from, but if the bees come after me, I'll be stuck, so I try harder with the trunk. *Shake. Shake.* Still no action.

I'm standing in the darkening yard, ready to give up, watching the stars come out one by one and, next, the fireflies, when I think of a rope. Back to the garage. This time, I actually do climb the tree. Hesitantly, I pull myself up. My knees are stiff and I fear falling.

Twenty years ago, climbing a small tree like this would have been easy. I was confident and strong, but I'm no longer used to trusting my muscles. Slowly, like an albino gorilla in my white suit, I pull myself along the slanting trunk until I can loop the cord around the branch the bees hang on. If this doesn't work, I'm giving up . . .

Back on the ground, I reposition the wooden box below the massive ball of bees and move to the side. I pull on the rope. *Shake. Shake.* Nothing. With more vigor now!

SHAKE!

Plop!

When the mass falls into my box, I'm so amazed, I just stand there . . . then, rousing myself, before the bees can escape, I slam the lid on my trap and jump back. Not all of the flying insects made it into the receptacle but most did. The stragglers will stay with the colony if I managed to capture the queen. I smile to myself.

It's been a long time since I've been forced, on my own, to cope with some physical challenge. Not since the farm . . .

When you have someone around as handy and talented as Tom Harman, you aren't often tested. Later tonight, my friend will come home. He will crawl into bed, exhausted from his long trip and the weight that he carries.

"I saved them," I'll whisper as he curls around me.

"What?"

"I rescued the swarm."

AQUARIUS

It's raining again, a steady gray drizzle, the wettest summer I can remember. The creeks rise over their banks. There's flooding in the
southern part of the state; whole trailers, all that families own, float
downstream like wood chips. The raging mountain rivers bring torrents
of muddy water into our lake, but at last the sun shines.

Mara and I sit in the gazebo looking down at the sparkling water
and watch two bluebirds court in the lilac bush. I was so surprised, this
afternoon, to see her as she came down the drive. Our friend's on her
way from Maryland to Berea College, in Kentucky, for a conference on
women's issues. She does this sometimes. Just shows up.

"I heard an interesting story the other day," I start up. "It made me
think about our homebirth days. You know there are more women
than ever choosing to deliver at home? The C-section rate in the U.S. is
over 33 percent, and the higher it gets, the more families will opt to stay
away from the knife.

"This was a wild one. I got this from my midwife friend, Rayne, in
Ohio. A doula, pregnant with her third baby, wanted to have a natural
birth. She'd had two previous cesareans. One for breech, pretty traumatic, and the other just because her OB said she had to. Apparently,
in her local hospital they don't allow vaginal births after a C-section,
otherwise she would have gone to the nurse-midwives there."

"Why wouldn't they let her try? They used to." Mara takes a sip of
her iced tea.

"It's an example of how malpractice insurance companies end up
calling the shots. They either refuse to insure a hospital that does
VBACs—vaginal birth after cesarean—or they make the restrictions so
difficult that providers and hospitals give it up.

"Anyway, this woman, Sophie, I think that's her name, contacted my
friend, Rayne. She's one of the few nurse-midwives who do homebirths
in Ohio. They came to an agreement, even though Rayne lived three
hours away.

"Last week, Sophie called after midnight to say her water had broken but nothing was happening so she was going to bed. She told

Rayne to go back to sleep, too, and she'd call her when contractions started. Rayne got up at dawn, packed up her birth stuff, and was already on her way when the pregnant woman called again, this time on the cell.

"'Where are you?' Sophie asked.

"'Two hours away, in the car, on the road to your house,'" Rayne told her. "'Are you in labor? Are you having contractions?'"

"'Yeah, they've started but they aren't bad yet,' the woman tells her. 'My husband is filling the portable birth tub. I figure the baby will come sometime this afternoon.'

"Rayne, the midwife, picks up her speed, but she isn't worried. Thirty minutes later her cell rings again. This time it's the husband.

"'How's she doing?' Rayne asks. She knew the man wouldn't be calling if his wife could talk, so it must be hard labor.

"'Where are you?' the guy demands— no 'Hi' or 'How you doing?'

"'Ninety minutes away. How's Sophie?'

"'Pretty cranky, and I'm worried. Contractions are getting close.'

"'Well, what's she doing? Is she in the birthing tub? Tell her to get out. It's too relaxing. Get her in bed on her left side to slow things down.'"

"Yeah, right," Mara interjects. "Slowing down a woman who's had three babies is like slowing down a semitruck coming down a mountain grade."

I nod agreement and go on with my tale. "'She won't!' the man says. 'She tells me the contractions will hurt like hell if she gets out!' He's all upset. Swearing and everything. 'If we'd gone to the hospital, this wouldn't have happened!'

"When you think about it, you can't blame the guy. His wife's been attending births as a doula for over two years. She's comfortable with the process. The only deliveries he's seen were in the operating room."

"So . . . ?" Mara says. "So what happened?"

"The next call Rayne gets, as she's hurtling down a narrow secondary road, is Sophie again. 'You can stop speeding,' the mother says. There's mellow music on the stereo in the background . . .

"Well, the cool thing is, the woman got her dream. She had her vaginal delivery after a cesarean section. She didn't mean to do it alone, but the baby came out. She caught it herself."

"Holy cow!" Mara exclaims. "What if something had happened?"

"You're right, but it didn't. She just put her hands under the water and held on, eased it out, first the head and then a gentle push for the shoulders, just a little grunt and then the whole body slipped into the water. She just flipped it over and let it float to the top. This is what Rayne told me . . . Just as it came to the surface the baby's eyes opened and they gazed into hers.

"They named the baby Aquarius."

"The dawning of Aquarius. The age of Aquarius . . . Remember that song?" Mara muses.

"Yeah . . . but can you picture it?" I take Mara's hand. "Sitting in the birthing tub looking into your infant's face, three inches under the surface? You'd have a minute or two. The newborn won't breathe when he's still in warm water and the placenta is attached and pulsing. Can you imagine? His little head is cradled in your hands. He scrunches up his face and then opens his eyes . . . luminous, holding all the wisdom of the ages . . ."

Lifeline

I'm in my office at home, answering e-mails on my silver laptop, when the phone rings and I run to answer. It's Zen calling on his cell from Camp Unalayee in the Cascades, near Shasta Mountain, the same Quaker wilderness camp for kids that Stacy and I worked at years ago. Since our youngest returned from Hawaii, he's called every week, and this is Sunday, his preferred day, so I take the portable out on the porch and prepare for a cozy chat.

"So, what's happening?" I'm expecting an answer like "Not much," but instead I hear . . .

"I was in a terrible automobile accident today."

"Yeah, right." I'm not alarmed, the kids like to jive me. "You're joking. I can tell."

"No, Mom. I wouldn't joke about this. Not about this."

He sounds so serious. I'm starting to believe him . . . "Are you OK?"
I figure he is, or someone else would be calling.

"Yeah . . . I'm OK. We were all taken to the emergency room in ambulances. There were four of us. We rolled three times on a mountain road in an SUV. There was blood everywhere. All the windows and doors were blown out. Joplin has fifty stitches in her leg. She and I were sitting in the back. We came out the best."

I don't want to ask, but I have to. "Did you have your seat belts on?" Ever since Tom was an EMT, we've always insisted our boys wear seat belts. Now that they're on their own, sometimes they do; sometimes they don't.

"Yeah, Mom. We all did. Dakota, Joplin's sister, was driving. The bones in one of her legs are shattered, but they think they can fix them. The other woman, Deidra, who was in the front passenger seat, has a broken neck . . ." A chill runs through me and I grab the porch rail.

"Deidra's in the operating room now. They took her first. They're putting a metal plate between two discs to try to stabilize the spinal cord. Her mom's flying down from Washington. Joplin's mom is flying up from Mendocino tonight."

He's talking like a clinician giving report, but I'm picturing the blood and the fear. The vehicle turning over and over. Bodies smashing against windows. Glass flying. I remember my accident in our first Volvo, the sound of the crash, the reverberation of metal splintering.

"You sound so calm. Did your life flash in front of you?"

"No, Mom. I knew I was going to be OK." I can hear him smile.

❄

Zen's near-fatal accident has shaken me the way Willow's death did years ago. How did he *know* he would be OK? It could have been the director of the camp calling from northern California, giving us the news that it was our son who had broken his neck . . . or worse.

Orion thinks I need therapy because I worry too much. When I was a flower child, think of the chances I took? But as you get older you see that there are real things to worry about. People die. Tragedy happens. Counseling won't cure that.

Orion in Ohio, Zen in California, and Mica in Russia. What kind of times are these that we all live so far apart? All a mother wants to do is keep her children safe, but how can I do that in a world with so much danger?

Zen and I hang up. I know Tom will call him when he gets home from the hospital. He'll want a full medical report.

A small brown fuzzy caterpillar catches my eye as it swings on a six-foot-long thread from the porch eaves. I notice that its black stripe is thick this year. Mrs. Shoepeck would say we'll have a hard winter.

The caterpillar is futilely trying to inch its way back to the roof on the delicate strand. I contemplate its fate, so vulnerable, clinging there. That's us, dangling from a lifeline, a filament that could break by a mere change in the breeze.

Fall

CHAPTER 7

Drums of War

"Hey, bud. I found something this morning." I look up briefly as Tom wanders into the living room, carefully taking off the long apron that Zen gave him; the southwestern design on the front nearly covered with clay. He's wearing his Bluetooth in his ear and I smile to myself. Once he was practically a Luddite, used only hand-powered tools; now he's a techie with earpiece and iPhone.

"I was searching through that old box of my journals and I came across this." I indicate a blue folder with a thick pink rubber band holding it together and a torn orange sticker on front that says FREE BOBBY. "It's yours. Want to see?"

My husband plops down next to me, picks up the file, and runs his fingers over the faded orange sticker. "Bobby Seale was one of the Chicago Seven, the leaders of the peace demonstration during the Democratic National Convention in Chicago."

"Well, listen . . . this touches me." I take the notebook back. "It's something you wrote. 'Refusing the draft was the most painful thing I ever did. My older brother was a soldier in the jungles of Vietnam. My parents, my pastor, even my Eagle Scout leader supported the war. Everyone thought I was crazy, or worse, *un-American*. The most unfortunate outcome was that in freeing myself from the war machine . . .'"

I stop to see if he's still with me. He stares out the corner windows but flicks his eyes to my face, so I read on. "'The most unfortunate outcome was I hurt my parents. I did violence to them, in the name of nonviolence . . .'"

When I pause I'm surprised to see that Tom's eyes are moist. I hadn't expected this sort of reaction. "You OK?"

"Yeah . . . I was just thinking about my mom and dad and how I wounded them. It still haunts me. You know how I thought about the

war, Pats . . . how *we all* thought. I couldn't fight there. When I burned
my draft card, my parents felt I'd betrayed everything they believed
in, everything they'd tried to teach me. Years later, my mom agreed
with me, said she saw how destructive it was for that country and for
ours . . ."

A twirl of golden leaves blows off the trees. I've known Tom the
man, but had forgotten, or maybe never knew, Tom the boy who left
his secure midwestern home, everything he grew up with, to create a
new world.

TV and movies portray hippies and protestors as kids going crazy
with love and drugs, but in reality there was pain everywhere. Pain, on
our families' parts, when they lost their children to a world they didn't
understand. And pain, on our part, when our parents rejected us for
not believing what they believed and not wanting to live as they lived.

Pain when we saw the photos of the war on TV. Pain when people
we loved were put in jail for protesting or killed as soldiers in the jungles
of Vietnam. We put flowers in our hair, partly to celebrate and partly
because we'd be too sad if we didn't.

※

As I'm putting away Tom's file in the box of old journals, a wrinkled
piece of paper flutters to the floor. It's a picture I tore from a magazine
over thirty years ago, and the war in Vietnam explodes into my office.
Shrapnel shatters the framed photographs of my family on the white
bookcases. The smell of napalm fills the air.

I remember this photo. It's of the naked Vietnamese girl, her mouth
open as she runs through the rubble of her village after a napalm attack, her face twisted in terror. In the background, American soldiers,
boys and men from *my* country, follow her with guns. You don't have
to understand the politics of imperialism to know this is wrong. You
don't have to be a midwife or somebody's mother to protest this with
all your heart.

I stare at this vision from the past. Where are the eloquent black-and-
white photos of Afghan children? Does the media take cues from the
Pentagon to shelter us from this war, or are the photos omitted because

the public doesn't want to see? What I'm thinking is . . . the drums of war *rumble,* but they're not roaring, like in the Vietnam days . . . . *or maybe I'm just not listening.*

When I glance out the window, the ghost of the little girl limps toward me across the grass. Only this time she's wearing a burka.

CHAPTER 8

JASMINE

When I enter Room 2, the lights are off. This surprises me, but in the gloom I catch sight of a young woman stretched out on the exam table.

"Hello. Are you OK? I'm going to turn on the lights now." The patient jerks up. She's a tall, thin girl with hair like a lion's mane, golden waves framing her face. A long paisley dress hangs over the guest chair and she's wearing the blue exam gown.

"Oh, gosh. I'm embarrassed. I thought I could catch a nap."

"That's OK." I glance at the front of the chart for a name. "Jasmine . . .

"I see that you had a positive pregnancy test. Are you happy about that?"

The girl shrugs. "Well, it's not what I planned, but my mom had me when she was fifteen, and I'm almost seventeen. You might remember her. Dawn Otterman? She comes to you."

"Dawn?" I calculate back seventeen years ago, when Tom and I ran the teen OB clinic at the university hospital. This is *baby* Jasmine.

Now that I think of it, she looks like her mother, same hair and dark almond eyes, only Dawn didn't have a chain of butterflies tattooed up her arm or a tiny nose ring.

"I delivered you!"

The patient grins. "I know."

I lower myself to my rolling stool. "So have you told your mom and dad about the pregnancy? Are they OK with it? Are you OK?"

"Yeah, sure. My mom wanted to come to my appointment today, but I said no. If I'm going to be a mother, I can't have my parents hauling me around . . . And Ryan's happy about it, too. He's the baby's daddy, a freshman at the U." When she says this, her face flushes. You can tell she's in love. "We'll probably get married at Christmas. It would help if I knew the due date. My periods are always irregular."

I do her exam and am surprised to discover that her little tummy is already rounding. Before she leaves, I give her the OB packet with her handouts on nutrition, weight gain, and exercise, then take her to the ultrasound room. "Want to see your baby?"

"Sure! Ryan will be so jealous! He wanted to come, but I said nothing would happen that he'd care to witness."

It takes me a few moments to find a nice view of the fetus. "Look, you can see arms and legs! He's waving at you."

"It's a girl," Jasmine says.

"You sound pretty sure of that."

"I had a dream and my mom predicts a girl, too."

Jasmine is already twelve weeks pregnant, so though I've just met her and would like to keep her with me for a few more visits, it's best to send her on to the midwives who will do her delivery. "Be sure and let me know when you have the baby," I call as she strides down the hallway, smiling at the photo of her unborn child. "I'll come over to the hospital to visit."

I picture the young woman's mother, Dawn, now a school principal with her master's degree. She's only thirty-two and she's going to be a grandma. It shows you that all teen pregnancies don't end tragically.

It's surprising that I can remember Jasmine's birth at all. There've been so many. I didn't want to tell my patient, but her mother was a terror in labor.

The fifteen-year-old arrived at the hospital in active labor, paced the room like a wildcat, and only allowed the nurse to monitor the baby's heart rate three times. Her mother and older sister just huddled against the wall and tried to keep out of the way.

Since she wouldn't let me examine her, I had to go by the sounds she made. High notes, active labor. Frantic notes, transition. Sudden drop to contralto, baby's coming! The universal birth song.

Dawn insisted on pushing while standing up. The nurse was freaked out. The attending OB, hearing all the commotion, stuck his head in the door and asked if I needed help.

"No thanks. I've got it under control." Ha! There was nothing I could do but glove up and hold on. The baby's head delivered into my hands, Dawn swung around, took hold of her wet crying infant, cord still intact, and plunked down on the bed.

"It's OK, Jasmine," she cooed. "It's OK." Then to me and her mother and the RN, she announced, "That wasn't so bad."

Now *baby Jasmine* is going to be a mother, and though she is only seventeen, the way she strides out of the clinic, confident, unafraid, I believe she'll be OK.

I remember the tattoo, chain of butterflies circling up her arm, spiral of life.

Shadow

"Hey, Tom, did you see the e-mail from West Virginia Patriots for Peace?" I'm coming out of my study. "There's going to be a demonstration at the courthouse in a few weeks. Want to go?"

"Nah."

Tom's slumped in the white canvas chair in the shadowy living room, staring out the corner windows. I suspect he's brooding about Gladys. As he expected, she's phoned to protest being fired. The nurses took the calls the first two times. After the third time, he spoke to her himself. True to his word, he didn't cave in.

"I'm sorry," he told the patient firmly. "Your drug screen was positive for cocaine and it says clearly in your narcotics contract that you'll be dismissed if it's discovered that you use street drugs." He didn't let her start begging. "Good luck with everything, Gladys. And have a good life." Then he hung up, but it cost him . . . *Another slice of compassion down the drain.*

"What's up?" I flop down in the matching white canvas chair next to him. In the dim light, it's hard to tell, but he seems to have a patch of eczema under his right eye, a sure sign he's under stress.

"Something else has happened at the office." I hold my silence. "Linda, at the front desk, was at her husband's company picnic and overheard two women talking in the ladies' room. The first said to the other, 'If you want narcotics, go see Dr. Harman. He's easy.' When Linda told me, I felt sick." Tom rubs his hand across his chin as if to wipe off something dirty.

"Did she say who the two women were? Where they're from?" I'm ready to defend him.

"Don't get so wired, Patsy. It's not your concern. That's why I almost didn't tell you. You are so *hyperreactive* and I don't want to deal with it." He jerks up, goes into his study.

What's going on? My husband doesn't usually shut me out like this. The frown line grows deeper above my eyes. Roscoe, our beagle-basset, pushes her head under my hand. I scratch her ears and wonder what will become of us. These rumors about Tom and narcotics hurt him. For over ten years he's been running our chronic-pelvic-pain clinic and he tries so hard to be cautious with the patients' medication. The women sign narcotics contracts, are given only long-acting meds that are hard to get high on. We do routine drug screens, even run a support group at our own expense . . .

Tom's walking away leaves a hole in me. I used to think we had a close family, but I can't say that anymore. The boys don't call. I haven't heard from any of them since Zen told us about the auto wreck two weeks ago. They don't e-mail, either, and now Tom withdraws.

Roscoe bumps my hand again. "It's just you and me, girl."

Witness

"Peace now!" a short fleshy man in a yellow raincoat yells through a megaphone. "Peace in the Middle East now!"

Crossing Clifton Street by the Mountain State Bank, I catch sight of the ragtag group of antiwar protesters, many with umbrellas like multicolored mushrooms. The group is gathered on the sidewalk in front of the three-story brick courthouse. It's been drizzling all day.

I'm disappointed that Tom wouldn't come. Inspired by reading what he wrote about the war in Vietnam and the photo that dropped out of the old journal, I asked him again to join me. It's been so long since we've done anything overtly political and I know he cares. Stacy, who lives with his wife, Sara Meretti, the donor of our first good Volvo, the one I totaled on the back roads of Roane County, will be demonstrating in Charleston, where they live now.

"Nah," Tom said. "You go ahead, I've got to put spouts on my teapots." Secretly, I was pissed.

I'm shy in this gathering, surprised that I don't know anyone here and unsure where to stand, with the older women in the back, holding signs that say GRANDMOTHERS FOR PEACE, or with the enthusiastic young people up front. I step up to the curb and nod at a purple-haired nymph with a nose ring. She holds a sign over her head that says HONK IF YOU'RE FOR PEACE.

The clock over the courthouse says 4:15 p.m. . . . I felt moved to come to this gathering, tired of being so politically passive, but now that I'm here alone, I'm uncomfortable. *I'll stay an hour and then I'll go home.*

A beat-up Suburu passes, with Trish, my friend from the Family Health Care Center, at the wheel. She gets excited when she sees me and almost runs onto the curb. The wispy purple-haired young woman next to me raises her sign, HONK IF YOU'RE FOR PEACE. Beep! Beep! Trish honks back. I wave and throw her a big smile.

More cars, vans, and trucks, with drivers of all ages, go by. They beep, toot, and blare their horns in support. I wave and holler, getting into the spirit. "No more war!" Then a slim, tanned young man wearing a tight tie-dyed T-shirt asks Purple Hair if he can give her a break and hold her sign for her. He smiles, revealing straight white teeth, takes the placard, and climbs up on a newsstand. Suddenly I feel like crying.

The guy has holes in the knees of his worn jeans, like Tom did thirty years ago, and though I don't find him nearly as handsome as the men I've loved, I know that to Purple Hair he's a hero.

Behind us, under the trees on the square, the grandmothers harmonize. *Peace, I ask of thee, oh river* . . . I'd like to sing, too, but if I opened my mouth, I would break down.

I wipe my eyes surreptitiously. Am I sad that in this university community there are only seventy-five people willing to stand up to the government? Am I lonely because Tom wouldn't come with me? Or am I moved, that even in these dark times there are a few souls who continue to witness for peace?

A small boy walks back and forth with a sign almost as big as he is. When Mica was three, he carried the same sign against his little shoulders. WAR IS NOT HEALTHY FOR CHILDREN AND OTHER LIVING THINGS.

We shall overcome, someone begins. *We shall overcome someday* . . . the crowd joins in, but I don't open my mouth. *Will we overcome? Can we? With the destruction of the rain forest, the economic meltdown, global warming, wars and rumors of wars around the world, the forces of ignorance seem more insidious than ever.* Once "We Shall Overcome" defined our generation. Now it's more like "We Will Survive."

CHAPTER 9

Beast

Early Saturday morning, Tom and I are startled awake by thunder. When we rise, we're surprised to see snow floating down like feathers. The sun flashes out, golden under the low slate clouds, then the thunder rumbles again. Strange weather for early November.

Tom hands me a mug of coffee and we park ourselves in our pajamas in the white canvas chairs. Leonard Cohen's "Waiting for the Miracle" is playing low on the stereo.

"Did you get the visa applications?" Tom asks.

"Yeah, I faxed them back and sent the passports yesterday. What a hassle. I had no idea it would be so hard to get into Russia. Think we really should go?"

Tom gives me his half smile. "The tickets are already paid for." He knows how lonely I've been for Mica and this is part of my Christmas gift.

We sip our coffee and watch as the brave nuthatches swoop down to the bird feeders but are scattered by bigger birds. "It's been weeks since we've seen a cardinal, where could they be?" I ask Tom. "I heard that, despite the weird early snow, this is the warmest fall on record. Are the birds as confused as we are?" I wait for an answer, not sure I'll get one.

"Maybe." Tom's a man of few words, but I chatter on . . .

"And yesterday I got an e-mail warning that bears have been sighted in Blue Rock Estates. Did you get it? A woman who lives at the outer edge of the development says she saw one rooting through her trashcan. Residents are warned not to leave their garbage out and to guard small children and pets." I repeat this last part with a snicker. "We live only ten miles outside of town. How could there be bears in Blue Rock Estates?"

Tom laughs. It's so good to hear his familiar chuckle. "People in this neighborhood get hysterical over the smallest thing . . . I've got to make rounds at the hospital. I'll be home in a couple of hours." He rises, pulls on his green L.L. Bean jacket, and goes out the front door. I smile to myself, thinking of a large hairy beast making its way though this affluent suburb.

It's not impossible; the black bear population in West Virginia is growing. If a bear really is close by, I know where he's headed . . . our beehives. I finger the silver Navaho bear, a talisman that I wear lately on a chain around my neck. If a bear is somewhere in Blue Rock Estates, he knows where I am.

JON

I'm on my way home from work and must stop as seven deer cross Blue Rock Drive, five adults and two fawns. They mosey over the medium unafraid. It gets like this in the autumn during hunting season. Here in Blue Rock Estates, a woodsy suburb where shooting is forbidden, we are overrun with flower- and shrub-eating varmints. You might as well have a sign at the stone entrance, DEER PARADISE.

It was late fall, just this time of year, that I began my clinical rotations in midwifery school twenty years ago. I had been apprehensive about how I'd fit in with the traditional university program, a hippie self-taught midwife who'd already delivered one hundred babies at home. Now the jig was up and I was in a huge tertiary monolith about to do my first hospital delivery.

"I'm going to take a smoke break," Mary Rose tells me as she leaves the labor room without warning. St. Paul Ramsey is a far cry from the cabins and farmhouses where I'd delivered babies before.

Mary Rose, my preceptor, is not what I'd expected. I'd hoped for someone sympathetic toward homebirth, but M.R. is a hard-bitten veteran who'd served in the military. I'm careful not to bring up the subject of her armed forces career. She'd probably been a nurse in Vietnam while I was picketing the draft board.

Our patient, twenty-one-year-old Carla Flores, a small, dark-haired girl with a belly the size of a watermelon, is in active labor and I'm wondering where her husband or mother is. Maybe she doesn't have one. I'm her family today, her sister, her mother, her midwife. It's Carla's first baby, and when we'd checked her an hour ago, she was five centimeters dilated.

The young mother keeps her eyes closed most of the time, no chitchat between contractions, and I honor that. She isn't like me. To deal with the pain of labor, I needed breathing patterns, back rubs, kinesthetic distraction, music, walking, bathing in water. All women cope differently.

"You all right, Carla? You look so beautiful and strong. Is there anything I can do?" I sit down on the one chair in the austere room, a hard-backed wooden rocker.

The girl cracks an eye. "Beautiful? I don't feel it."

"Is there *anything* I can do? Rub your back, massage your feet?"

"You'd do that? Rub my feet? Would it help?"

"Maybe a little."

"OK."

☿

For thirty minutes, as I stand at the end of the hospital bed massaging Carla's little rough feet, I stare at the mountains and hills running along the fetal-monitor strip. Once I would have been gazing through windows of a cabin at the lush green hills of West Virginia. I hum a lullaby under my breath. *To my little one's bedside in the night . . . comes a new little goat, snowy white.* The song may or may not soothe my patient, but it soothes me.

Carla moans.

"You doing OK?"

She shakes her head no. "It's my back!"

Great, I think. *Back labor.* "Do you want to get out of bed?"

"Can I?"

I step to the door and look up the empty corridor. There are no nurses around. I don't know what the rules are in this inner-city hospital. I guess it's all right. *We're midwives, for God's sake!*

I turn off the fetal monitor, help Carla step into her slippers, and assist her to the bathroom. "Sit here for a while. If you lean forward, it takes the pressure off your back." I show her how to open her legs and bend down until her head is almost between her knees. "Do you want me to stay here and rub your back?"

Carla gets that faraway look in her eye as another contraction comes on. "No, I'll be all right. I need to go to the toilet."

Her calm amazes me. At this point, many women would have asked for pain medicine. I retreat to the birthing room, an old OR suite, and straighten the sheets. The walls are cream tile, but the nurse-midwives have made an effort to make the space seem more homey. There are framed pastoral landscapes on the walls, and the hospital bed has a flowered quilt. This is the first birthing room at St. Paul Ramsey and it's clearly an afterthought, an attempt to keep up with the fancier hospitals.

There's another moan from the bathroom. *Where is my preceptor, anyway? I hope she didn't forget about me.* I step into the hall and look out again. An intern in blue scrubs nods as he hurries by.

Behind me, in the john, I hear a low growl and I turn to skid across the linoleum. "Carla! Don't push."

"I'm not pushing. The baby's pushing!"

"Well, don't help it. Go like this. Hoo! Hoo! Hoo!" I show her what I mean as I guide her to the bed and tip her over on her side. "No pushing. Just blow. It may not be time yet."

Who am I kidding? Of course it's time. The sound of that grunt is universal. With one hand I reach for the call light and press the red button; with the other I grab a pair of exam gloves. Carla's eyes are wide open.

"Hoo! Hoo! Hoo!"

Mary Rose jogs into the room and takes in the scene with a glance. "What the hell? Why didn't you call me?"

I already have my fingers in the patient's vagina. "Fully dilated and plus one station," I report. "I didn't know she was progressing. She was so calm; the contractions didn't seem very strong. I got her up to the bathroom and—"

"You got her up to the bathroom without doing a vaginal exam first?!" M.R. scolds.

"Ughhhh," Carla yells and I feel the baby move down another inch.

"Well, get ready, for God's sake!" That's Mary Rose.

I slide the girl up but take time to touch her face. "It's going to be OK."

My instructor drags a delivery table over. I pull my sterile gloves off and remove the end of the bed so that the woman's bottom is right on the edge.

"Gown!" she commands, holding out a sterile surgical robe backward. I'd helped the physicians on with theirs many times but fumble as I stick my arms into the sleeves.

"Now gloves," M.R. orders like a drill sergeant, nodding at a new pair opened on the bedside table.

"Hoo. Hoo. Hoo. Hoo. Hoo!" I encourage Carla.

The instructor, also gloved and gowned, kicks the rolling stool over and nudges me to sit down.

We both take two deep breaths.

"We're ready now, honey," Mary Rose says softly to Carla, her first gentle words, and I see another side to her. "You can push."

Toward *me*, M.R.'s not so gentle. She grabs my hands in hers and holds them over the baby's head. From somewhere, an RN appears, replaces the monitor belts and sets up the infant warmer and oxygen.

Beep . . . beep . . . beep . . . . . . beep . . . . beep. The fetal heart rate is decelerating, but it's just head compression. This baby will be out in two minutes. I try to give the fetal scalp a tickle to speed up the heartbeat, but my mentor's hands are glued over mine.

Carla lets out a long yell and curls forward.

"That's the way, honey! Hold your breath as long as you can while I count," the RN instructs. "One thousand one. One thousand two. One thousand three."

There's too many cooks cooking this stew. Carla's doing fine, just as she is, without the RN's help.

If we were at home in her bedroom, I'd be putting olive oil on her perineum right now. I look over at the gleaming silver instruments arranged in rows on the sterile delivery table, half expecting to see a little cup of mineral oil, but of course it's not there.

Beep . . . . beep . . . . beep . . . . beep.
M.R. lets go of my hands and reaches for a pair of scissors.

At first I assume she's getting ready to cut the cord, though the
head's not out yet, but she nudges me with her elbow and forces the
scissors into my hand, then injects Xylocaine into our young patient's
perineum. Now I know what she wants me to do . . . cut an episiotomy.

So here I sit. The head of a dark-haired infant crowning before me.
I know how to get this baby out without a laceration or episiotomy in
two minutes, if Mary Rose and the enthusiastic nurse would leave me
alone, but I am *the student,* enrolled to learn.

I take the scissors and cut, feel the skin crunch between the blades,
see the blood ooze . . . and deliver the baby. It's not a good feeling, but
it's done. The very pink body swivels out, Mary Rose cuts the cord, and
the RN takes the tiny boy to the infant warmer.

"If the heart rate's down, you have to cut an episiotomy right away,"
Mary Rose whispers. "The OBs watch us, and if you hesitate, they'll
start coming in to every delivery to supervise." She looks at the door.
"We don't want that."

"My baby. My baby," Carla cries.

"Everything all right?" a balding OB asks, peeking in from the hall.

"Fine," Mary Rose and the nurse answer together.

It isn't until we're done stitching and have the new mother cleaned
up that Carla gets to hold her tiny one. "Jon," she calls him, with tears
in her eyes.

Just then there's a knock at the door and a thin young man in jeans
and a West Point T-shirt comes in. "I got here as fast as I could."

Carla looks up and there are tears for real now. She holds out the
baby. "Your son," she says simply, as if introducing a prince. The father
kneels at the bedside, glances at the baby, takes his woman's head in his
hands, and holds it to his heart.

"Thank you," he says.

So this is Carla's rock, her hero. When her eyes were closed and she
was so quiet during the hard contractions, he's the one who was holding
her hand, as Tom and Stacy once did for me. Behind her eyelids this is
the partner that stood whispering, "You can do it. You can do it."

Mary Rose and I don't say a word, but she wipes her eyes and I realize that she's crying. She takes my hand. We are both crying . . .

♉

The deer make it over to the golf course on the other side of the road and wander down the hill. I stop at the mailbox and pick up the mail. There's a letter reminding me that it's time to renew my membership in the American College of Nurse-Midwives.

Most people think all midwives do is deliver babies. They don't know that some are employed by family-planning clinics, some teach in universities, and some, like me, work in women's health practices doing prenatal visits and gyn. As I gather my briefcase and pocketbook, my water bottle and scarf, I mull over my day. It's not that all the patient encounters had the intensity of birth . . .

Haala, nineteen, from Saudi Arabia, is expecting her first child. She doesn't speak English, has never had a pelvic exam, and is scared to death. Her husband, an engineering student at the university, must translate every word I say. She sits on the exam table, her arms closed around her chest, wearing the regulation blue exam gown, her burka still covering her head. I use my hands and my smile to communicate and finally make her laugh . . .

Martha, forty-five, is getting divorced; she cries when she tells me how she found out that her husband of twenty-five years cheated on her with a coworker, a woman Martha had actually befriended. Her mascara is running. I roll my exam stool closer and wipe her wet face with the back of my hand . . .

Priscilla, fifty-one, has a sixty-year-old husband, a retired coal miner, who's unable to have sex. He refuses to discuss his problem with his doctor. I ask Priscilla if she's ever tried a vibrator, and give her a handout showing where to order small tasteful devices. We giggle like girls . . .

I support these women, praise them, teach them, like any midwife would do for a pregnant patient. I tell the women that they are beautiful and strong, the same way I did when Carla was giving birth . . . but these women are giving birth to themselves.

Winter

CHAPTER 10

Homecoming

Tom and I have returned from our long-planned trip to Moscow, a beautiful city of marble subways and Russian Orthodox cathedrals with golden domes. Rose can hear now, with her little bone-conduction hearing aid that she wears on a crocheted headband like a miniature hippie. And this time when I sang her to sleep, I know she heard my lullaby. It helped my feelings of separation just to sit on the sofa with Mica, my little blond boy, now a big man. We held hands like we used to when he was two and we walked through the Minnesota woods.

�֍

Back at work, we discover that the staff has decorated the office for Christmas. An artificial fir tree, covered with silver and mauve ornaments, sits in the corner of the waiting room. Silver snowflakes, each one bearing the name of a staff member or provider, hang from the ceiling.

The first thing I hear when I hit my desk is that Ruby, our pelvic-pain patient, is pregnant. Her chart is on top of my stack with a message to call her.

"Hi Ruby, this is Patsy Harman, nurse-midwife. What's up?"

"Oh Patsy, I'm glad it's you. I don't feel so good today."

"My nurse, Abby, told me you came in and had a positive pregnancy test. She says you're about five weeks along and she set you up for a new OB visit. *How* don't you feel good?"

"My stomach, my lower stomach. I'm cramping. Oh, Patsy. I'm afraid I'm gonna miscarry."

"Are you spotting?"

"No."

"Have you made love lately?"

250

"Yeah, just this morning. Could that make me miscarry?"

"No, Ruby. Intercourse doesn't cause miscarriages, but it could cause your endometriosis to flare up. Why don't you just rest today? If you start bleeding or the pain gets worse, you should go to the ER. I really think things will be OK. Next week when you come in we'll have to start weaning you off your narcotics. Did the nurse tell you that? They're not good for your baby?"

"So, I'm *not* going to miscarry?"

"Ruby, I don't know for sure, but since you aren't spotting, I don't think so. Just rest, OK? And come to the ER if you begin to bleed . . . There's nothing we can do for a miscarriage anyway. No way to stop it, but I bet you'll be OK." I say my good-byes and get off the line, then flip through the rest of the charts.

Fifty percent of the calls we get are from the chronic-pelvic-pain patients, who represent only 5 percent of our practice. Some of the women are manipulative, wanting more narcotics. Some just need reassurance. Some may be having a true emergency. You have to really listen to sort it all out . . .

Ruby's been on narcotics for three years. She started them when she was waiting for surgery and afterward, when she was no better, continued. It will be hard to get the young woman off, but we'll step down gradually. Stopping suddenly would cause both the mother and fetus to go into withdrawal.

At least Ruby will be motivated. She wants this baby, and she has a nice boyfriend. Abby says he came in with her for the pregnancy test, a good-looking blond, a lineman for Mountaineer Electric. The two sat in the waiting room with their arms around each other, so excited they outshone the Christmas tree. Though the baby is less than a half-inch long, it already fills their hearts.

Winter Solstice

Winter has locked around us for sure now. As I leave from work, the storm begins. Snow coming in from the west. By the time I get to the freeway, the tops of the mountains are covered with white.

Despite a recent bout of melancholy, I'm excited. I always love the first good snow, and it's winter solstice night. "Hello snow!" I greet the lacy clumps that whirl from the low gray clouds. It's going to be a big one! They're predicting eight inches.

Oh, the weather outside is frightful . . . I sing along with the radio.

On Turkey Run, the shortcut behind the University Agricultural Farm, the traffic slows and I find myself thinking of Ruby. I saw her in the clinic this afternoon for her first OB visit. Six weeks is early to start prenatal care, but that's fine with me. I like to see the women as soon as they call, talk to them about how to have a healthy pregnancy, answer their questions, get lab work, and go over their history for risk factors. Despite her spotting, on the early ultrasound we could see the fetal heart flicker.

❦

I hand Ruby a thick green folder with our Women's Health Center logo printed on the front, a pine tree with the slogan, "Take care of yourself. Your health is a valuable resource."

"What's this?" Ruby asks.

"These are your OB handouts. You don't have to read them all tonight." I make a little joke of it.

There are hundreds of books on childbirth, but in our practice the patients' educational and socioeconomic levels vary so much . . . some women have their PhDs . . . others never finished high school. Some have read *Spiritual Midwifery* and *The Working Woman's Pregnancy Book* before they come for their first visit; others don't read at all. For this reason, I like to start the educational process early.

I remove the flyer titled *What to Eat for a Healthy Pregnancy* out of the packet and place it in Ruby's lap. "So what did you have for breakfast this morning?"

"I don't usually eat breakfast. No appetite." She shrugs as if that's the end of it. But I don't give up easy.

"I know what you mean. Me neither. But when you're pregnant that has to change. So what *could* you eat? Do you like milk?"

Ruby and I problem-solve together on healthy food choices, things that are handy and not hard to cook. I have to be careful in my suggestions, because Ruby is on a medical card and doesn't have much money. I tell her how to get signed up for WIC, the federal program that gives pregnant and nursing mothers coupons for free healthy food. Ruby still smokes a half-pack of cigarettes a day, has limited understanding of nutrition, is underweight, doesn't exercise because of her chronic pain, is unmarried, with a lot of family problems, and is still on narcotics. This will be a challenge, but I like challenges, and I like Ruby.

❀

Once I'm on the freeway the traffic thins out, but at the top of our steep drive, I stop singing. If the snow gets too deep, I won't be able to get my Civic back up. I take a deep breath and drive down anyway. *Let it snow. Let it snow. Let it snow . . .*

Since returning from Moscow, I've been lonely for my boys and have had a hard time getting into the holiday spirit. I managed to get a tree up, a wreath on the door, and the manger scene laid out, but that was the end of it.

Inside, I toss my briefcase in my office and shake off the blues. Soon Zen will be home . . . we haven't seen him for six months . . . and Orion and Ari and Lissie and baby Abraham will be here for Christmas.

Though it's still afternoon, I put on an album of seasonal music and scurry around the house collecting candles for our solstice ceremony. This year, as last, it will be just the two of us. I glance out the window where snow now blows in at an angle, thankful that I made it home early. The gazebo is already covered, and six inches of fluff coats the porch rail. If the roads get too bad, it might be just me.

A blast of wind jolts the house and the lights go off. The microwave beeps. The stereo goes off. When I check the telephone, there's no service. When I flip open my cell to call Tom, there's no connection. No refrigerator sound, no fan from the heater. *No heat,* I remember. Even though we have a gas furnace and gas fireplace, electricity controls the pilot.

It's nearly dark now and from the corner windows I can no longer see the oaks twenty feet in front of the house. I light one of our old kerosene lamps we brought from the farm. The wind slams the other side of the house and the whole building shudders. I've been in storms like this before, in Minnesota and at the commune. You'd think I'd be afraid, but I'm strangely excited.

⚺

"Whoo! Whoo!" Someone calls from out on the porch. I hurry to the front door. When I pull it open, white swirls in.

His arms are full of groceries. His L.L. Bean jacket and hair are plastered with snow.

"Happy solstice!" It's Tom.

In twenty minutes, the two of us are seated at the dining room table. The room is dark except for the circle of yellow from the kerosene lamp. I can almost imagine the fragrance of wood smoke from a cast-iron cookstove and can see our little boys, Mica, Orion, and Zen, sitting with us.

Tom strikes a match to light the first taper. "This yellow one is for the sun, giver of life." Then it's my turn. "This gold candle is for family." We take turns saying prayers.

"This pink one is for little kids." I picture Rose, Abraham, and Lissie.

"The white one is for love." I look in Tom's eyes and am so grateful to be here with him as the blizzard rages around us.

I glance at the candlelight flickering on the ceiling. The wind still howls in the trees out front. "I love the house in this light. Wouldn't you like to live with kerosene and candlelight always, maybe in a little log cabin?"

"We tried that before, Pats, remember?"

"Oh, yeah! How could I forget." I laugh at myself and we keep lighting candles until they're all gone.

"This one is for change, the only constant."

"This one's for the earth."

"This one is for the yet unborn." I think of Ruby and her baby.

Grace

Christmas morning, in the dim light before dawn, I lie in bed determined to appreciate my blessings. I miss Mica and his family but I must trust them to lead their own lives. For a few minutes, I lie in the dark, sending light and love their way and to my brother Darren and my mother, gone now to where mothers go when they lay their burdens down. Then I sneak out of bed to fill the stockings. Outside the corner window, the snow flies again.

Soon, we are opening presents. Orion and Zen look like true Soviets in the leather and sheepskin hats that Mica bargained for at the Moscow open-air market. Everyone tries hard to keep baby Abraham from ripping open all the packages, but it's a losing battle. In the middle of everything Mica calls and we pass the phone around. "How you doing, man?" "What's up, dude?" "Did you open your presents yet?" "How'd you like those caps?"

By eleven, the living room is an ocean of gift wrap and the sun comes out. Handel's *Messiah* plays on the stereo. *Every valley shall be exalted, and every mountain and hill made low; the crooked straight and the rough places plain . . .*

❦

In the kitchen, while I'm toasting bagels for brunch, I peek around the corner to watch Zen playing cards with Lissie, and Orion rocking little Abraham gently against his chest. What good and gentle men they are. Not perfect, but good . . . *The only prayer we need is . . . thank you.*

I remember when baby Abraham was born, I thought to myself, a new soul has entered the universe and everything must shift over, the trees and the sky, the rocks and the stars. Even my heart must open wider, for one more joy, perhaps one more sorrow.

CHAPTER 11

Fall from Grace

"So, how was your day?" I ask as Tom settles himself in front of the fireplace.

"OK."

He's not too talkative, but I make up for that. We slouch on the sofa, sock feet up on the coffee table. It's a chilly night, and the wind blasts the front windows.

"I saw Ruby again this afternoon," I offer. "You know she's expecting. I'm weaning her off the narcotics. She's happy about being pregnant, and I think she's going to be OK." I glance at my husband, who stares blankly at his reflection in the dark windows. "You tired?"

"Yeah, I am. I did six surgeries at Community Hospital today, but it's not that . . . Dr. Parsons took me aside in the doctor's lounge. She told me that her husband, who's an internist at the University Hospital, says the physicians over there are saying I'm the 'go-to guy' if a woman in town wants narcotics."

I squint like hot water was thrown in my face. This is an insult to Tom, to our whole practice. We've tried so hard to run the chronic-pelvic-pain clinic professionally, providing a counselor for the support group at our own expense, Xeroxing each prescription so a patient is unable to alter it, insisting patients not get narcotic scripts from other medical providers. This is *worse* than when Linda heard the druggies talking about Dr. Harman in the women's restroom. These physicians are Tom's colleagues and peers.

"Why would they say that?" My voice goes up in outrage.

"I don't know. They're primary-care docs. They probably see our patients at the walk-in clinics or the ER and notice how many are on narcotics. They don't know all that we do in the office to prevent misuse of the meds."

My husband lets out a long sigh that reminds me of Zen . . . "What bothers me most," he goes on, "is that the University Hospital has no chronic-pelvic-pain program at all. Well, the Anesthesia Department has the Pain Center, but all they want to do is teach residents how to do nerve blocks. I know what disdain they have for our patients. They think they're all druggies, faking their ailments. But I've seen the insides of the women's bodies during surgery; rarely is there a normal pelvis."

My husband slides down farther on the sofa and I pull his head into my lap. Tom loves to be touched, probably more than anyone I know, but for some reason there's not been much touching lately. I stroke his hair and his shoulders. He closes his eyes.

"Want to go to bed?" I mean more than sleep and I'm not usually so bold.

"I'm beat, Pats. It's been a long day." *This is not like Tom. I offer sex and he turns it down?*

"Can I just sleep here?" He looks up at me pitifully with a half smile that reminds me of that time long ago when he was so sick in the butterfly tent.

"You want me to just sit up here all night, holding your head?"

"Yeah," my friend answers, almost in dreamland.

"Like that's gonna happen!"

I run my fingers through his short silver hair and sing him a lullaby. *My bed is too small for my tiredness* . . . He is so weary from the cares of the world . . .

It has been fifteen years since we were part of the teaching faculty in the Department of Obstetrics and Gynecology. We came straight from Cleveland, where Tom did his residency at Case Western Reserve, full of natural-childbirth zeal. I was the first midwife in labor and delivery in recent memory and did my deliveries sitting on the side of the bed, without a mask. The women were allowed in the shower and were monitored only periodically. Tom was the only doc who let his patients use a squat bar and didn't cut episiotomies. We started an OB teen clinic.

The trouble is, we were too successful. Soon, hundreds of women in town who wanted a natural birth were seeing us for prenatal care.

Unable to sacrifice them to the roulette wheel of academic practice, we volunteered to come in for their deliveries.

"We're working so hard, it's like we're in private practice," Tom observed. "Maybe we should be." The idea grew and in time we went out on our own to create the Women's Health Center, the kind of medical environment in which we believed, where women were always treated with respect.

I continue to stroke my lover's head, the best backup doc a midwife ever had . . . *Wind, blow the moon out . . . please . . .*

CHAPTER 12

RIVER

Light shining through ice. A cloudless blue sky. Snow under my feet. It's been weeks since we've heard from the boys, and their silence worries me. Tom says quit fretting. Let it be.

Determined to do as he tells me, and singing under my breath, I pack a lunch of rice crackers and cheese. *Let it be. Let it beeee. Seeking words of wisdom* . . . I grab my parka and car keys and head for Swallow Falls State Park in the higher mountains.

❦

As I wander the snow-packed trails, an announcement stapled to a worn wooden bulletin board attracts my attention. "Caution, Hikers: Bears have been observed in the park. Do not approach them. Do not feed them." *Bears again,* I think, fingering my silver bear ornament. I wouldn't mind seeing one. Hard to believe they would come into this busy recreation area.

At the fall's edge, a man and a woman lean against a rail, arms around each other, staring at the cascade of frozen water. The yellows and blues glow from within like a rippled sheet of opal. They nuzzle each other, and I find myself wishing again that Tom were with me.

I miss my lover. I asked him to come, but he stayed at home to do pottery. Maybe it's just as well. Being alone in nature always brings me peace, brings my shattered heart together.

"Hey, slow down there!" a father yells. Two little boys run ahead of their parents, skidding on the ice, just like Orion and Zen did when they were that age. I miss them too . . . It's funny. I didn't have empty nest when they first left home after high school. Tom and I were actually thrilled to have the house to ourselves. We were dancing around.

"No more worrying about curfews or the boys getting in trouble!" It's only now, when I realize they're not coming back, that I long for them.

A group of young adults in colorful parkas, with lift tags attached to their zippers, cross my snowy path. These are not the bulky Appalachians I'm used to seeing at Shop 'n Save or Walmart. These are athletes who come to the mountains for rock climbing, whitewater rafting, hiking, and skiing. I wonder if, despite the beauty around us, they realize that Wild and Wonderful West Virginia is one of the most polluted states in the nation.

I stop to take photographs of hemlocks in the perfect slanting light, recalling Laurel's e-mail of this morning. "Did you know that *Forbes* magazine ranks West Virginia fiftieth in terms of the greenest states? Number fifty, *dead last* and who else is at the bottom? The same states that are the worst in every other index of poverty and health."

The article she attached contained a picture of a mud-swollen West Virginia stream. The caption said we have the fourth-worst scores in water cleanliness and more toxic waste to manage per capita than all but three other states, Mississippi, Louisiana, and Alabama.

I kneel in the snow next to a small ice-covered creek to take a shot of the shadows and light, wondering if it's the industry in cities such as Charleston, Huntington, and Wheeling that cause the problems, or the coal-powered electric plants like the one on the outskirts of my town. Probably all of them.

Coal is King in West Virginia, and a hunger for commerce controls the decision makers at the capitol. Few people in the state, rich or poor, are concerned about global climate change or the carbon footprint that coal leaves. What they care about is their paycheck to put food on the table or their corporate profits. Need, greed, and shortsightedness leaves a beautiful region contaminated.

※

Listening to the water bubble under the ice, I follow the little creek down to the roaring river. Two men in wetsuits and helmets carrying kayaks pass me, heading for a small icy beach. The shore is covered with glistening pebbles, and they slip and slide as they get to the water. "Having fun?" I ask, surprised to see them out in the cold.

"You bet," the shorter guy, with a straight nose and a strong jaw, grins. Not a bad-looking man, with a little ponytail. He reminds me of Tom when we first started doing homebirths.

Before Tom went to medical school, he'd delivered only two babies, Orion and River. I can't remember how he happened to get his hands involved in River's birth.

Penny and Kevin, from the food co-op in Spencer, were our good friends. Maybe Tom wanted to practice doing another delivery, since he was a new EMT. Whatever the reason, Penny was easygoing, calm and in control. This was her third baby.

For the first time, our roles were reversed. I poured olive oil over *Tom's* fingers and handed *him* warm compresses. Penny pushed, while Kev supported her back. In her own home, in her own bed, she gave birth to an eleven-pound baby, vaginally, without lacerations, the biggest infant that either of has delivered to this day. Tom still brags about it.

As I watch from the rocky ledge at the side of the trail, the men settle themselves in the low boats, one red, one blue. The breathtaking whitewater rages over boulders, catches the light in the spray. Where the spray hits the rocks it adds to the ice, but most of the water moves too fast to freeze.

The guys ready their paddles, then expertly maneuver their tiny boats into the current, catch the rapids, and race away. I laugh and clap my hands like my five-year-old granddaughter, Lissie. The men are so beautiful and brave. The kayaks get smaller and smaller, until they disappear where the majestic, possibly toxic, river turns north.

Games

Tom is quiet this Sunday, a cement pallor just under his skin. I haven't seen him like this since three years ago when his patient, Dottie Teresi, a neurologist's wife, suffered a post-op complication and was in the ICU for two months. The dime-sized patch of eczema on his cheek is the size of a quarter, and he plays a computer game on his laptop while he waits for a call from the hospital. *Not a good sign.* When Tom withdraws into computer games, you know he's stressed out. Now and then he stops to chew his cuticles.

It's clear he doesn't want to talk, but I break into his game anyway. "Jasmine came into the office today to show off her belly. She's almost due. Remember when her mother, Dawn Otterman, had her baby? That was a scene!" Tom doesn't answer, doesn't even smile. He stands up and stretches his back.

"What's happening, Tom? Is something wrong?"

"It's Bobbie Boyd. She's the pelvic-pain patient that had that bleeding problem after surgery and I had to take her back to the OR. She came into the Emergency Department in the middle of the night for abdominal pain, distention, and fever.

"It's been months since I operated on her, but she identified me as her doctor so now I have to go see her. What I dread is running into her husband again. I just hope her problem doesn't require surgery." Abruptly he shuts his computer, rises, and strides into the bedroom, emerging in shorts, a Presidente beer T-shirt from the Dominican Republic, and his weight-lifting gloves. "I'm going to the gym."

"Why don't you call the ER first, see if they've got Bobbie's flat-plate X-ray back? It's their move, right?"

"Patsy, lay off! I'm the doctor here. This isn't a game. I'm going into the hospital after I work out. I'll take care of it." He stalks out the door. I recognize his anger about my medical suggestions; this is a spark, not the full conflagration.

Tom is less resilient than he used to be. He's grinding his teeth at night, and the dentist says he needs expensive crowns. The fear of being sued troubles us both. We cringe at each surgical setback, wait for a blow.

Seventy-five percent of ob-gyns in the United States have been named in lawsuits. And midwives, who used to never be sued, are also hauled into court. The last student midwife I mentored has already been a defendant, and I *know* she was good.

Tom used to say that the threat of being sued was the cost of doing business in health care, but since he was named in a frivolous claim last year and the insurance company settled, we wonder if that cost is too high.

I flash back to when we lay under the full moon, near the fountain on the Ohio University campus. How innocent we were in our desire to serve the people. We had no concept of the forces that would be against us, medical-malpractice insurance companies, difficult patients, the rising costs of running a practice, shrinking reimbursements, lawyers out for a few million bucks.

Outside the window, Hope Lake sparkles, ever changing, one day jade green, one day turquoise, the next day slate, or khaki, or shit brown. Today it's shit brown.

❧

Two hours later my cell phone chirps. It's Tom. "I'm on my way home," he announces. "I just left the hospital."

"That was quick." I picture the color returning to his face, starting pink at the neck and rising.

"I think Bobbie's just constipated. The X-ray showed her bowel's full of stool. We gave her an enema. She's resting comfortably now and her CBC is normal. The fever was only from dehydration."

"Want to have a glass of wine with me when you get home?" I try one more time. Tom knows the code.

"Maybe a nap, Pats. After the ER called last night, I didn't sleep well."

"All right." My heart creeps a little farther into its cave. This is the second time he's turned me down. Outside the corner windows, five crows have moved into the big oak by the water and they flap, like black shadows, across the yard.

Cord around the Neck

"You go on," I yell, signaling my husband to pass me. It makes me nervous when he rides my tail. He speeds by on his royal blue recumbent, the BMW of low-rider bikes.

I have the bike trail to myself this afternoon, no hikers, no joggers, and no mothers pushing strollers. It's our first ride in many months, and the green river moves placidly along at my side. It was three years ago that this waterway flooded and, in a rage after a fight with Tom, I took a night ride through the middle of a lightning storm . . . *near death by stupidity.*

Already bluebells, white bloodroot, and yellow starflowers cover the forest floor. The air is alive with birdsong, and I stop in the middle of the trail when I see trilliums, beautiful trilliums, early this year.

My reflections are cut off as I catch sight of Tom coming back toward me. We pause to share a bottle of water. As he slugs back a drink, his cell phone goes off. "Shit. I've been paged twice since we started, two different pelvic-pain patients. One was Gladys, begging me for more narcotics. I told her she had been dismissed and I couldn't help her. She should go to the ER.

"The other was Ruby. When I tried to call her back, her line was busy. That pissed me off. This cell phone is driving me crazy. It feels like a goddamned cord around my neck."

Tom isn't usually so cranky. "Here, give me your phone. I'll take the calls."

"Thanks." He takes a big breath and lets it out slowly. "I shouldn't let it get to me." Then he pedals off and I punch in the saved number.

"Hi Ruby. This is Patsy Harman, taking the emergency calls. How can I help you?" I emphasize the word *emergency* so the patients won't call just to chat.

"Oh, Patsy. I'm glad it's you. I'm cramping again. My pain is real bad today. I know you said I need to wean off the narcotics, and I've been trying, but I just can't make it on two pills a day. Do you think you could call in some more Percocet, so I could take three? And maybe give me one more Duragesic patch? They used to work good." I go on alert when she mentions *cramping*. This isn't an ordinary chronic-pelvic-pain patient. Ruby is pregnant.

"Cramping, like menstrual pain?"

"Yeah, like my period . . . only real bad. *Real* bad, Patsy. Worse than before."

"Any bleeding?"

"No, just pain."

"Did you have intercourse?"

"Not this time."

"When did you poop last?" I glance around to see if anyone's passing. *I'm talking about poop in public, for God's sake.*

"Couple of days ago. Can you get me a few more patches?" The woman is persistent.

"No, Ruby. That isn't going to happen. I can't give you any more narcotics. It wouldn't be good for the baby. We have to keep to the schedule. In fact, we'll be stepping down further next week. You need to get your bowels moving. This is a common problem in pregnancy, and it's worse for you because narcotics slow the motility down. After you get emptied, if the pain is still bad, you'll have to go to the ER. They'll examine you and call us. Can you go get some Metamucil or a stool softener? Can you do that?"

"I don't have a car." Ruby is whining like a six-year-old and I see why Tom gets irritated.

"Well, call your stepmom or someone."

"They're all gone to the mall."

"Do they have cell phones?"

"Yeah . . ."

"Well?"

"*OK!*" This is said in a teenage-like huff. "But the Metamucil *probably* won't help . . . If I *try* and I'm still in pain will you call in a prescription for some Oxycontin?"

"*No, Ruby.* We can't take a chance with the baby and we can't go back up with the narcotics. You'll manage OK. Get someone to come home and sit with you. Partly you're afraid because you're alone. "

"I guess." Ruby disconnects without saying good-bye and I step down on the pedals. Tom is already far ahead. I can just see the red and yellow dot of his bike shirt rounding the bend.

That wasn't my best moment as a midwife. I was really rather harsh, but Ruby is going to be a mom. She needs to understand the personal sacrifices she'll be making.

I flash on something I've said to myself more than once: *It hurts to be a mother. It hurts to give birth and it can hurt a lot more later* . . .

Spring Again

CHAPTER 13

Blame

Spring comes in a rush to Appalachia. One day you notice tiny buds on the plum tree and the next, I'm not kidding, the whole tree is a bouquet of pink. The forsythia blaze and daffodils march along the front walk, but when I get to work, the clinic feels muted and strained. I'd like to find out what's going on, but my schedule is overbooked and I'm way too busy to investigate.

The first thing I see when I get to my desk is a note from Dawn Otterman, Jasmine's mother, that her teenage daughter has delivered a seven-pound baby without pain medication and has already been discharged from the Birthing Center. It was a girl, as they'd predicted. I take time to send them a card.

Along with the usual prenatal visits, menopause problems, early OB visits, yeast infections, and annual exams, I see a twenty-one-year-old woman, Dannie, who wants to become a man. We have a long talk. Once a transgender patient would have shaken me, but after we helped a previous patient, Kasmar, successfully make the transition, my mind is more open.

By four, I'm at my desk attacking a two-foot-tall stack of charts. Across the hall, I hear the name *Ruby* mentioned in a low voice by one of the nurses, and I briefly wonder if it's Ruby Tuesday, my OB patient, but go back to my tasks. Within an hour the office is empty. No one even stops by my door to say good-bye.

As I review and sign my last lab report, I dial Tom's cell. "Hey, where are you? You up for a bike ride?"

"Just down the hall." I smile to hear his voice from both the receiver and the other side of the clinic.

"I haven't seen you all afternoon. I thought you were in the OR."

"No, I came back to the office an hour ago."

"So, you want to go riding?"

"Nah, Pats. I don't feel like it. You heard what happened . . ."

"No . . . What . . ."

"Come over here; I don't want to talk about it on the phone." This sounds serious. I snap the cell shut and take the shortcut through the lab.

"What? What's up?"

My partner leans forward on his desk, Beatles tie pulled loose from his shirt collar. He runs his hands over his head and across his face. "It's Ruby. She's dead."

I back away from him. "Pregnant Ruby?" I know very well whom he means; I just don't want to believe it. He nods.

"But I just talked to her a few days ago. I told her to go to the ER if her pain got worse. She wasn't bleeding or anything. What happened . . . ?" I'm thinking of a pulmonary embolism or maybe a blood clot in her groin.

"Dr. Wheaton called from the University Hospital ER. He's pretty sure it was a drug overdose. Her body's been sent to Pittsburgh for an autopsy." My husband pushes a chair toward me and I fall into it. "But I just *talked* to her. I told her we couldn't give her more narcotics. We were weaning her off . . . She can't be dead. Was it my fault? I just talked to her . . ."

"No. You did the right thing." We look at each other, both wondering what the repercussions will be. Will the coroner call for an investigation? Will the state Board of Medicine get involved? But mostly we're just sad for Ruby, silly, selfish, once alive, beautiful Ruby.

Somewhere far out to sea, Tom and I bob alone, up and down, on the lead gray waves.

Silence

Breathe in. Breathe out. I'm sleeping alone again, in Zen's old room, and the worry about Tom curls around me like snakes. Since Ruby died, he isn't himself. Neither of us are . . . but we can't comfort each other.

My husband comes home later and plays video games longer. We never make love. Yesterday I saw he'd left his wedding ring in the bathroom, and when I asked him about it, he said his hands were swelling. It crossed my mind that he could be having an affair. There is silence between us. The silence is cold.

Earlier tonight, lying in bed with him, getting ready to read a chapter of a mystery together, I tried talking, thinking that if he could express what's bothering him, he might feel better.

"These last few months have been hard," I begin obliquely. "I've been worried about morale at the office, the staff aren't getting along, and the boys never call . . . There's just been so much going on with the chronic-pain patients, and now Ruby . . ." I want to take off my armor, tell him I'm also concerned about *us,* about our relationship. He cuts me off at the first sentence.

"You stick your nose into other people's business too much, Pats. That's your problem."

There's silence again, this time from me. *Screw you,* I think, and snap the silver vest plates back across my chest.

"Maybe I'll go downstairs and sleep in Zen's old room."

"No you won't." Tom grabs my arm hard. "Let's read." And so we do, and my blaze of resentment banks into coals.

In the night, for the third time in two weeks, I move downstairs anyway.

Breathe in and breathe out, I tell myself. *Stop thinking. Stop picking at your worry and grief and guilt. It spreads into your soul like poison.* Just breathe and find your calm center.

❧

In the deep night I wake, dreaming of Ruby and Aran. Aran was my friend Trish's daughter. The nineteen-year-old died when she was only a few months postpartum, another narcotics overdose; this one by street drugs. Tom had delivered her baby. I was her midwife. I should have known she was in trouble . . .

In the dream, it is storming. Aran and Ruby are calling for me from an old rusted car down by the lake. By the time I get there, the car is under water.

CHAPTER 14

Circle

Eleven strong women sit in a bright contemporary living room near Shepherdstown, West Virginia, discussing the state of childbirth in the United States. This is over on the Eastern Panhandle, where Pennsylvania, Virginia, Maryland, and West Virginia all come together in a tangle so confusing you wonder if the surveyor, maybe George Washington, might have been drunk.

The women in this circle come in all shapes and sizes. Most are dressed in slacks and sweaters. The grandmother next to me, with frizzy gray hair that sticks out around her head like a halo, wears an elegant brocade jacket that I especially admire. The young midwife across the room, with a seventeen-month-old baby, sports a blue T-shirt that says MIDWIVES HELP PEOPLE OUT.

We eleven represent the rest of the fifty nurse-midwives in the state. The others are at home today . . . birthing babies, or on call, waiting for babies.

In this circle of midwives, some work in large groups, some in small, some with state agencies, some with ob-gyns, some with family docs. A few of us own our own practices, but more are employed by hospitals or physicians. Only one of us doesn't deliver babies: me. What we have in common is a passion for treating women with respect and a devotion to childbirth as a normal physiological event, not a disease.

"My goal," says Gerri, a small woman with straight short hair who sits against the wall on an ottoman, "is simply for my patients to have the kind of birth they want." Her voice is soft and her eyes luminous.

I think about that as I stare out the floor-to-ceiling windows, across the sunny high plateau toward the Appalachian Mountains. Not every woman does get—even with a midwife like Gerri at her side—the birth she wants . . . That would be, let's face it, a two-hour painless labor with our loved ones around us, no episiotomy, a vagina that immediately goes back to shape, breasts that spurt milk, and no postpartum depression. But I know what Gerri means. She wants to support the women wholeheartedly in their goals. Again, it comes down to respect.

"I had a patient the other day," I tell the group, "who asked me if I thought any of the docs in town would support her in having a C-section without labor. It took me aback because I'm very much against C-section on demand, but for the first time, I wondered if she had a point.

"She was a skinny little thing, thirty-five years old. Weighed about ninety pounds, with hips like a twelve-year-old boy. Her sister had had one of those labors where she lay for three days . . ." The group laughs.

"Why is it always *three days?*" Nicki asks. "Never four or two days . . . it's always the same. It's like they all had the same labor!"

I smile, raising my eyebrows. Nicki's right . . . It's always *three days.*

"Anyway," I go on, "she told me about her sis and I went over the risks of cesarean section, how it's major surgery. Even in the best of hands, there are dangers . . . infection, hemorrhage, and, rarely, death. I asked her how many children she wanted and explained that the scar tissue after C-sections can lead to pelvic pain, more miscarriages, and even increased incidence of fetal loss . . . but she only wants one baby and then wants her tubes tied.

"I looked at her little bony body and thought . . . maybe she has a point. It might make sense, but I told her to wait until the end of her pregnancy and make a decision with her doctor and midwife. If the head is really low and the baby is small, she should give it a shot."

The conversation drifts to health-care reform and how badly we need it in West Virginia. What I'd really like to talk about is Ruby's death, how it has affected Tom and me, but something holds me back. Maybe I'm afraid of litigation, maybe I believe we should have known the repercussions when we started the pelvic-pain clinic and the narcotics program . . . maybe I just sense that these women, who deal with the happy part of midwifery, wouldn't understand what it's like to wonder if you are responsible for the death of a mother.

We hear updates from each practice, go over our new chapter by-laws, and eat pie. Then the sun, stretching low on the carpet, tells us it's time to go home. Before the women gather their things, I ask that we hold hands.

"Thank you for reminding us," Shona says. "When you aren't here, it doesn't feel the same." This surprises me. *Why wouldn't it feel the same? Is it possible I bring something special to the group, something from the days when talking to trees and prayer were what you needed to get by?*

We rise and I send love through my hands . . . into these other hands . . . that will touch women . . . that will comfort . . . that will birth joy.

Step by Step

One wrong turn and twenty minutes circumnavigating in a wide circle and we're back on 68, heading straight into the setting sun, toward central West Virginia. The Great Sleeping Bear of the Appalachians rises before us, then the mountains close around.

Shona, Nicki, and I are each thinking our own thoughts as we come down the Allegheny Ridge, past the lights of the Hazelton federal prison, that place of heartache that reminds me of a fairy castle. A CD of women's music plays low on the stereo and I'm trying to pick out the lyrics. *Step by step we're heading in the right direction,* the vocalist sings. You can take this line in more than one way.

I think of myself as a person of faith, but I sometimes wonder. So many things seem to be going wrong . . . First there's the state of obstetrics. Somehow, in my simple mind, the warping of childbirth seems connected to what we've done to the earth.

Then there's the death of Ruby.

And finally my marriage. Tom seems so far away. Fog closes around me.

Step by step . . . the woman sings in her clear soprano. *Step by step,* the chorus repeats. Are we? Are we headed in the right direction?

Renunciation

It takes four to six weeks to get the results of an autopsy back. Four to six weeks if you're lucky, sometimes lots longer. Not that there's anything lucky about an autopsy . . .

Tom and I are on our way home from Hueston Woods State Park, in Ohio, where we rented a cabin and spent a long-planned pre-Easter weekend with Orion and his family. We dyed eggs and had an Easter egg hunt with the grandkids. We fed tame deer, played on the swings, and went swimming in the indoor lodge pool. We tried to act normal but the gold of daffodils and the yellow of the forsythia meant nothing. Ruby's death hangs over us.

I'm almost asleep when Tom clears his throat and says into the dark car, "I got the autopsy report back Friday."

"You got it." I sit straight up. "Why didn't you say so?"

"I didn't want to spoil your weekend. I know how you get."

I'm not sure I'm grateful, but maybe he's right. "Well . . ."

"Ruby's death was a clear overdose of narcotics. All the drugs in her body were meds I prescribed for her. She must have been stockpiling them. She had methadone and Lorcet in her bloodstream, two Duragesic patches on her arm and one in her mouth."

"In her mouth?" Somehow this shocks me more than the rest. "Why would she do that? Was she *trying* to kill herself?"

"The pathologist doesn't think so. There's no suicide note and he says that it's a method druggies use to get high. He's seen it a lot in the tri-state area."

I reach over and put my hand on Tom's leg. "Do you think it was because I wouldn't give her more meds? . . . No, that doesn't make sense . . . She *had* meds or got them somewhere . . . But she was five months pregnant! She had a tiny baby inside her and a nice boyfriend. He seemed nice, anyway. Maybe he partied with drugs, too."

I blink back my tears as we pass the gas refinery, the chimney belching blue flame. Ruby Tuesday wasn't my friend. Sometimes I didn't even like her. She was stubborn, childish, and self-centered, but she was also full of life. Now she's gone.

"I don't understand . . . why would she *do* that?"

"We'll never know. Most likely an accident. She was probably using her meds to get high all along. Maybe she had pain too; I know when I did her surgeries she was full of endometriosis . . . You think a patient's legit. You listen to her symptoms, respect her, try to help her, and this happens . . ." We drive in silence as we take the new bypass around Ohio University in Athens, then Tom speaks again.

"I just can't do it anymore, Pats. It's been eating away at me until nothing's left but a deep hole that I'm about to drop through. I've given all I can to the chronic-pelvic-pain patients. There are other women who need me. If I keep this up, I'll leave medicine altogether.

"At any rate, I've made a decision; I'm going to write all the doctors in town that I won't give narcotics to patients anymore except right after their surgeries. I can't be responsible for shit like this. People say I'm the go-to guy for narcotics? Well, the patients can find other go-to physicians, drive two hours to Pittsburgh or pester the ER docs, but it can't be me."

Helping women with pelvic pain has been Tom's specialty for the last fifteen years. Maybe he was naive when he started. Perhaps the physicians who refuse to give care to chronic-pain patients are right. You step into that role and something dark pulls you down. Narcotics are a tricky business, a godsend for many, a chain around the neck for others. Tom's been concerned about the patients' misuse of narcotics in the past, but I've never heard him talk like this before.

"And next week, I'm also going to send all the chronic-pelvic-pain patients a registered letter saying that they should begin weaning off their narcotics or find another care provider who will prescribe them. I'll see them all for another few months to give them time to get settled, but that's it."

"You could do that?"

"I *will* do that. They can come to us for routine gyn and other problems, but no more methadone or Oxycontin, Duragesic patches or Percocet. The women I feel worst about are the people like Cindy Carlton, the teacher. I feel bad for her and women like her who always use their meds as prescribed, never ask for more. It doesn't seem fair, but if I'm going to get out of narcotic supervision, I can't pick and choose. Let's face it; we've been fooled before."

We ride the rest of the way in silence, down Route 50, across the bridge at Parkersburg, and then across Route 68.

The moon is just setting when we pull down the drive. Four deer stand near the pear trees, now covered with blossoms. Tom stops the car, rolls down the window, and whistles once. "I could train these deer, I bet, if I whistled and threw them a pear." He grins and his eyes crinkle at the corners. For a minute, I think I see my old friend again, but maybe not.

Encounter

It's Saturday morning and Tom and I are biking up the trail along Ten Mile Creek. We don't talk much about Ruby Tuesday. We're both trying hard to get over her death, and the letters have gone out to the pelvic-pain patients. Below us, in the wooded ravine, the creek roars downhill over boulders as big as Rachel's old cabin. As usual Tom rides on ahead, pedaling hard.

Three vultures, circling low, catch my eye in a gap between the trees. Their wide fringed wings curl up at the ends, and they're so close I can see the individual feathers. There are vultures over Hope Lake, too, not just a few as in other years but scores at any time, circling, floating on air currents.

And it's rained every day for a month. Sun in the morning, by afternoon the sky is full of towering thunderheads, puffy dark clouds that extend from the horizon halfway up the sky. I've never seen anything like them. It's been so wet, I've had to replant the beans in the garden, twice. The seeds rot in the wet soil.

My mind wanders to climate change, again. Global warming isn't something we anticipated in the 1970s. We knew the black smoke bellowing out of the power plant down by Lake Superior was bad for our lungs, but never dreamed it could destroy our whole ecosystem.

I pedal on, admiring the pink and white phlox that fringe the gravel bike path. This world of ours is so beautiful. I'm in love with the flowers, the cascading water, the infinite variety of insects and animals and birds. Each season that comes and goes, I'm more aware of the colors, the light. I'm attached to every living thing and don't want to lose them, the clouds too, even the ominous, magnificent, towering thunderheads.

Movement catches my eye on the uphill side of the path and I stop my bike. Tom is long gone, halfway up the mountain, and it's fine with me. I thought once he'd made the decision to give up the chronic-pelvic-pain program he might be his old self again, but most of the time silence stretches between us, and we're just going through the motions of marriage. I step off my bike, stand very still, and crane my neck, expecting to see a fox or maybe a raccoon.

On the rocky slope, between the dark trunks of trees, mostly fir and hemlocks with a few maple and oak, I focus on a shadow. Did it move? As my pupils adjust, I see two black eyes, close set and surrounded by very black fur, looking back at me. *A bear stands on her hind legs not forty feet off the trail.* What's a bear doing here? They are usually far up in the mountains.

"Hello," I say in a shaky voice, trying to sound friendly. *You don't want to show fear at a time like this.*

The bear snuffs and scrapes her paw in the leaves. *Is that a baby bear in the rocks behind her?* The huge animal wags its head and snuffs again.

I'm not sure if the snuff is a greeting or warning, but I can't stay around to find out. Bears can run 30 to 40 mph when enraged. Cautiously, keeping my eyes on hers, I swing my leg over the bike.

The bear wags its head then drops to all fours, poised to pursue. I put my right foot up on the pedal. The bear makes a *whoosh* noise . . . I step down, my legs shaking, and move out with my head low over the handlebars, hoping to catch up with Tom. I don't look back, just push as hard as I can. It isn't until I'm a mile up the hill that I stop to rest. When I turn around, my lungs burning, there's no dark beast chasing after me, no friendly bear, or curious bear, or angry bear, just my fear.

CHAPTER 15

AKILAH

"You don't remember me, do you?"

The auditorium of the convention center in Boston is filled with nurse-midwives, several thousand, I estimate. Like songbirds, they come in all varieties. Peacocks, dressed in expensive summer suits with peep-toe wedges. Cardinals, in long paisley skirts and Birkenstocks. Wrens, in jeans and running shoes. One woman sitting in front of me wears a pink T-shirt that reads on the back, WE HAVE A SECRET. IT'S NOT THAT BIRTH IS PAINFUL, BUT THAT WOMEN ARE STRONG.

I sit toward the back of the huge hall, alone, at the annual conference of the American College of Nurse-Midwives. I wanted Tom to come, just for the experience, but he wasn't up for it. None of the other midwives from West Virginia came either. They're probably too busy delivering babies.

The woman sitting next to me, who looks to be in her late thirties, dressed in slacks, with an embroidered wool vest and long dangling beaded earrings, smiles and asks again, "You don't remember me do you? It's been a long time. You delivered my first baby when I was fifteen. I'm Serena. Serena Holt."

I study the coffee-colored face and brown eyes. "Was this in Cleveland?" My first official paying job as a midwife was at Case Western University Hospital, where Tom did his ob-gyn residency.

The session has ended and the auditorium empties. "Yes, at Case. I was a single fifteen-year-old mother and you took care of me in labor and then helped me give birth naturally. I have two kids now. The one you delivered just started college. The other is still in high school."

"I'm trying to remember. There have been thousands of births. Tell me something about your labor."

"Well, it was a long one. My water broke at 3:00 a.m. and I came to the hospital with my grandmother. My folks had all but disowned me. Kicked me out when I told them I was pregnant, called me a tramp. I was living with Gram, but she had to work. She'd just gotten on with the Board of Ed and couldn't afford a day off. My water was leaking, but I wasn't having hard contractions yet, still in latent phase.

"You sat with me all day, a scared kid, all alone. You entertained me with stories of the hippie days and how you became a midwife. You told me about other young girls like me, who'd gone on to college and made something of themselves. I've always remembered this one thing you said . . . I often use the same words with my patients:

"Labor is like playing cards. You don't get to choose the hand you're dealt. You just play the game the best you can . . . Life's like that, too.

"Anyway, once the contractions finally kicked in, I went fast. My grandmother made it back to the hospital and then my parents showed up. You wouldn't let them in the birthing room until after the baby was born, said it would distract me, that I had to concentrate on getting my job done. The baby was posterior and my back hurt like hell, but you got me through.

"That day changed my life. I named my little boy Akilah. It means 'wise.' You believed in me when no one else did, and here I am." She dips her head and passes her hands in front of her body as if introducing someone rare and beautiful.

"I finished high school, started community college, went into nursing, got my master's degree, and became a nurse-midwife because of you. When I was an RN in labor and delivery at Case Western University Hospital, we nurses used to tell stories about you after you left, funny things you did with the patients. We called you the wisewoman."

"The *wisewoman?*" I almost choke. In many countries the title *midwife* means wisewoman, but I am a child staggering through life. I wipe the corner of my eye and give my fellow midwife a hug. Life is a journey and you never know whose life you may touch.

Sacrament

A crow calls from the top of a maple. I lie on my back feeling the moss on the huge flat boulder under my palms. *I have been lost before, and come into these woods . . .* I remember the song I wrote on the commune such a long time ago . . . *to lay my burdens down.*

Tom and I are picnicking in the woods, in an empty campground, on the huge slab of sandstone surrounded by trillium at the state park. I open my eyes and catch my husband's profile as he eats his cheese sandwich. Good appetite I see . . .

He stares into the forest of hemlock spruce and a few hardwoods. The pink buds of mountain laurel are poised to unfold, and the forest smells of dirt and new growing things, but there is no celebration. We've been so estranged lately.

Sadness festers like a purple bruise just below my breastbone. Ours was a shining, forever love; in my heart a holy golden circle of light . . . and now . . . the candle flickers, about to go out.

I take a big breath . . . "Tom, what's wrong? I thought maybe once you gave up the chronic-pelvic-pain program you'd feel better . . . but nothing's really changed. There's dead space between us . . ." I roll over and tentatively put my hand on his leg. He continues to wolf down his sandwich and then swigs from a bottle of water. It's so quiet; I notice the wind in the top of the spruce trees.

Finally he answers. "I've been really down. It's everything. You want me to be the optimist, always cheerful and confident. You want me to buoy you up. When anything goes wrong, you expect me to hold it together . . . But I get tired of it." He turns and pushes my long bangs off my forehead.

I shake his fingers away. *It's true. I need him to tell me that all is well with the universe. That's his job! I rely on him . . .*

"It started after I got a letter from a law firm in Charleston about Bobbie Boyd; remember her, the bleeder I had to take back to the OR and her husband was pissed? I had a feeling the family would sue. Now they're saying she has lasting pain after surgery and the husband's lost the comfort of 'conjugal relations.' It's bullshit; she had pain when she first saw me, but the lawsuit isn't going to disappear."

"Another medical-malpractice claim?" A ripple of dread goes through me. This isn't the first time, but that only makes it worse.

"I didn't tell you about it because you get so freaked out. Anyway, it may have been anger about the lawsuit; I get so tired of this crap. You try your best to take care of patients and this is what you get . . . Or it could have been grief after losing my mom or hearing the other docs say I was the 'go-to guy' for narcotics, but I couldn't shake a feeling of gloom, such a weight I could hardly push myself out of bed in the morning. And then there was Ruby . . ."

I stare at my husband, a stranger despite his familiar face. He looks past me into the sky, where high cumulus clouds ride the wind.

"It was easier to deal with my depression alone than to have my problems compounded by your anxiety . . ."

I am stunned. Is this the same man I fell in love with, the same easy-going hippie bass player? And is this *me* he describes? The hyper, fearful, unsupportive wife, once a brave flower child?

"I'm better now," he goes on in a quiet, thoughtful voice. "Little by little . . . I never thought of myself as a person who could be so knocked off-kilter. I thought I was stronger. I thought I was immune . . ." He snorts a short laugh, "Shows you no one is . . ."

I throw my arms around him, hold on tight, and bury my face in his shoulder. "Tom, don't go away again." My lover presses his forehead against mine and kisses me, his lips warm and familiar, then my tears come for real. "You are my touchstone, even when you're unhappy. I don't want to drive you away by being so anxious."

When he rolls on my body, there's a buzzing in my abdomen, a buzzing like bees getting ready to swarm. The ground rises up, and we find a place far away from our troubles. The months of hurt roll back, like thunderclouds passing over the mountains. Storms will come again, I know this, but for now the sky clears and we are back under the Trillium Stone, skin to skin, heart to heart. In this place there is comfort and, in the end, light.

Hold On

A huge V of geese flies low over the water and lands on the bay. We're in the side yard of our house on Pelee Island, our first trip of the season, to ready the cottage for renters. The tall lilac bushes along the property line are blooming, and their scent fills the air. No moon yet. One by one, stars come out in the violet sky, and Tom and I vie with each other to see the next one. We've been singing old peace songs around a campfire. *Will every man 'neath his vine and fig tree live in peace and unafraid . . .*

How primitive we humans are, with our warring tribes, still thinking we can solve the world's problems of supply and demand with weapons, swords, spears, and bombs. I stare at the flames, flickering orange and green. It's my turn to pick a song.

"You, know," I say to Tom, "I can't sing 'We Shall Overcome' anymore, did I tell you? I used to think I had the answers, knew how to make the world better. All we had to do was *start a revolution.* Now I feel so confused and I guess I don't think we *can* overcome." I throw him a small smile.

My husband shrugs and tosses another log on the campfire. The flames shoot up and illuminate his face. "Did you really think we would *overcome,* Pats?"

"Yeah . . . . didn't you? I thought if men and women stood together for what was right, we would win. Like Gandhi . . ." I study my friend. "Didn't you?"

Tom kicks the chunk of wood farther into the fire. "I don't know. Maybe it doesn't matter. It's like the great mandala."

I hear the song in my mind. *Take your place on the Great Mandala.*

He goes on. "We just find our place on the wheel of life and do our best. To overcome won't take one generation, but many . . ." The waves slosh up under the break wall and pull away.

"I've been thinking, too," he says. "I'd like to invest in an energy-efficient heat pump at home and solar panels for the roof of the house. Maybe a wind generator up here at the island. I know it's not much, but maybe we could get some other people in Blue Rock Estates interested in alternative energy. We need another ten-year plan."

My head snaps up. "You mean like when we left the farm?"

"'Bout time for another one, don't you think?" Tom grins his old grin.

"Maybe this year we could invest in a hybrid car," I add tentatively. "Or maybe we shouldn't . . . The economy's still a disaster, we better hold off."

Tom gives my hand a squeeze. "No, we should move ahead. Nothing will change if everyone waits. Forget that saving the earth doesn't seem possible in the time required. We just need to do what we can. If it's not possible, we'll find out later." He pulls out a small notepad from the back of his jeans, crouches forward in the firelight, and begins to write. I lean on him, watching.

First the heading: New Ten-Year Plan. Then,

Energy-efficient heater at home
Wind generator at the cottage
Solar panels
Hybrid car

"I'd like to volunteer for more international medical missions too. What else?" he asks.

Once again we plow into dreams and timelines. We're a different Tom and Patsy than thirty years ago, but in some essential way the same. It isn't what's on the list that matters, but that we're moving forward.

It's a dark night. No moon yet and the Milky Way spreads across the sky.

"OK." I take a big breath, tentatively getting into the spirit. "We should shop locally. Use the farmer's market for vegetables that we don't grow and find someone who lives out in the country where we could buy eggs and meat if we want . . . or go back to being vegetarians . . . That's doable, isn't it? And you've been talking about volunteering for Doctors Without Borders. We should both go. You could do surgery and I could run a women's clinic, maybe teach local midwives, or deliver babies in a refugee camp."

Tom continues to take notes as the flames die down and then flare up again. The page fills and he flips it over and starts on the back. Finally he reclines in his lawn chair . . . and surprises me when he starts to sing "Paul and Silas." I join in, staring up at the stars, the same stars that shone over the campfire in Minnesota and on the communal ridge. This time we make it to the third verse. *Now the only thing that we did was right was the day we started to fight.*

This is a song I can sing with conviction.

I get it now. It doesn't matter if we overcome, we just have to take it, step by step, and keep our eyes on the prize. I belt out the song at the top of my lungs. Tom flicks me a look to remind me that we have neighbors. I laugh and sing louder.

Keep your eye on the prize. Hold on!

Hallelujah

The habit of wakefulness is hard to forgo. At 1:00 a.m., on Pelee Island, it's no different. I still pad through the dark living room, go out and inspect the sky like I do almost every night. The scent of the lilacs is calling me.

When I step on the narrow side porch, I draw in my breath. The full moon, like a new silver dollar, a circle of light, is just rising over Lake Erie and our beach towels and swimsuits twist on the clothesline like ghosts in the wind. Moon shadows, I think. Like in the Cat Stevens song. Leaping and hopping.

I reenter the bedroom and shake my husband on the shoulder. "Tom." He's hard to wake up. I shake him again. "Tom . . ."

"What?" he finally responds, sitting upright, not sure where he is.

"Come on. You have to see this. It's the full moon." I pull back his covers. "Come, *please.* You don't need to get dressed." Tom swings his feet over the edge of the bed and rises slowly, rubbing his eyes.

"What?" he asks again.

"You'll see." I lead him through the shadowy rooms, open the screen door, and push him out on the side porch in front of me. He stands running his hands through his hair and then peers around.

"Look, *moon shadows!* There's light everywhere, coming down from the bright sky and reflecting up from the huge body of water. It's magical."

Long silhouettes of the willow and maple and hackberry lean across the lawn. A stiff breeze comes in from the south and the willow leaves rattle. I take Tom's hand and we cross the dew-covered grass in our bare feet and climb the stairs to the deck on the break wall.

"Look, you can see clumps of sea grass, it's so bright. And the stones under water!" I pull off my pajama top. Tom takes in my white breasts. *He's back to his old self,* I can tell. I pull up Tom's shirt too and put my arms around him, chest to chest.

"Come on. Let's go swimming," I beg. "No one can see us. It's not safe if I swim alone . . ."

Tom grins. "I'll guard you from here." He knows that the shallow sandy South Bay stretches for almost a quarter of a mile before it's up to our chins; not much risk of a swimming accident. The waves roll in against the rocks like molten silver. I step out of my pajama bottoms and pad down the wooden steps.

"Come on," I plead again, looking back over my shoulder, wiggling my butt. "It will be fun!" Then I plow through the water toward the full moon. When I'm up to my thighs, I plunge in, holding my breath as long as I can, my eyes closed, letting the bubbles out of my mouth until the air's gone. The lake is cold, but just enough to make me shiver and soon I'm used to it.

I hear a splash and look back. Tom is running naked through the water, his head thrown back, laughing. When he catches up, I open my legs and hold onto him like a koala bear. We are swimming in silver and Lake Erie stretches for miles as smooth as gray silk. Above, it's so light that the stars are invisible, yet I know they exist . . . And there is music.

I begin to hum Beethoven's "Ode to Joy" from the Ninth Symphony. Tom picks up the tune and we hum in two-part harmony, floating on our backs, in the healing liquid, holding hands, far from shore.

"Look," I say. "When your eyes are just above the water, the reflection of the moon leads right to you, a river of light." Tom ducks his head like I do. "Do you see it?" I spread wide my arms. "This is our church."

Tom is still humming. Now he picks out the words. *Joyful, joyful, we adore thee . . . God of glory, Lord of love . . .*

He's on his feet and turns, moving slowly back toward shore, his hands outstretched, caressing the water with his fingertips. "I'm going inside; you coming?"

"Not yet. Soon . . . It's so beautiful . . ."

⚜

Joyful. Joyful. There is music like prayer, a prayer with one word. *Hallelujah.* These songs lift me up and at the same time bring me to my knees. I watch Tom, already climbing the wooden steps to the deck. I'm alone in the silver moon water, all alone on the little planet we call Earth.

It comes to me, then, that the caterpillar I saw at home, dangling by a thin filament in the wind, the day Zen almost got killed in the auto wreck, probably inched his way back to the roof.

Ruby Tuesday is gone but Zen is alive, and it might have been otherwise. We thought Rose couldn't hear, but she has a baby hearing aid and will learn to talk and to sing.

Joyful. Joyful. We adore thee. Field and forest, vale and mountain, flowery meadow, flashing sea . . . Teach us how to love each other. Tom and I are together again and the moonlight spreads out across the water.

For a long time I float on my back with my arms wide open, letting the silver liquid hold me, reflecting on my life as a midwife. What a gift it has been to me, a long journey, not yet over. Jasmine came to the office to show off her newborn baby, Karma, last week. The tiny girl was wearing tie-dyed cloth diapers.

I picture my boys, grown men, each on his own journey, slipping and sliding over the rocks, sometimes making a wrong turn, then finding their way again. Will they wake some moonlit night and go skinny-dipping?

I think of my grandchildren, growing up in this dark world.

I'm not a wise woman . . . but I must remember . . . to lead them into the water.

ACKNOWLEDGEMENTS

I'd like to thank those who made *Arms Wide Open* possible: My writing consultant, Dorothy Walls, for her encouragement. My agent, Barbara Braun, and her team, for their faith in the message. My editor, Helene Atwan, and the hardworking professionals at Beacon Press, for their commitment to publishing books that are real, true, and beautiful.

❧

I'd also like to thank my staff at our women's clinic for their support; my boys, who have allowed me to share pieces of our family life . . . and finally my husband, Tom, the best back-up doctor a midwife ever had.

❧

Arms Wide Open is dedicated to the women and men who taught me what it is to be brave and to all idealists who try, in their own way, to make the world better. We can never do enough, but we can try.

❧

And finally to you Dear Reader, I send a message: *Do not give up hope. In these difficult times the sun still rises, there is light on the water, and the full moon shines, once a month, in the dark sky.*